Ichthyoses

Current Problems in Dermatology

Vol. 39

Series Editor

Peter Itin Basel

Peter M. Elias San Francisco, Calif.
Mary L. Williams San Francisco, Calif.
Debra Crumrine San Francisco, Calif.
Matthias Schmuth Innsbruck

Ichthyoses

Clinical, Biochemical, Pathogenic and Diagnostic Assessment

89 figures, 15 in color, and 9 tables, 2010

KARGER Basel · Freiburg · Paris · London · New York · Bangalore · Bangkok · Shanghai · Singapore · Tokyo · Sydney

Current Problems in Dermatology

Peter M. Elias
Dermatology Service (190)
VA Medical Center
4150 Clement Street
San Francisco, CA 94121/USA

Mary L. Williams
Clinical Professor of Dermatology and Pediatrics
University of California, San Francisco
1700 Divisadero Street
San Francisco, CA 94143/USA

Debra Crumrine
Dermatology Service (190)
VA Medical Center
4150 Clement Street
San Francisco, CA 94121/USA

Matthias Schmuth
Professor and Chairman
Department of Dermatology
Innsbruck Medical University
Anichstrasse 35
A-6020 Innsbruck/Austria

Library of Congress Cataloging-in-Publication Data

Ichthyoses : clinical, biochemical, pathogenic, and diagnostic assessment / Peter M. Elias ... [et al.].
p. ; cm. -- (Current problems in dermatology, ISSN 1421-5721 ; v. 39)
Includes bibliographical references and index.
ISBN 978-3-8055-9394-6 (hard cover : alk. paper) -- ISBN 978-3-8055-9395-3 (e-ISBN)
1. Ichthyosis. I. Elias, Peter M. II. Series: Current problems in dermatology ; v. 39. 1421-5721
[DNLM: 1. Ichthyosis--diagnosis. 2. Ichthyosis--genetics. 3. Ichthyosis--pathology. 4. Skin Diseases--diagnosis. 5. Skin Diseases--genetics. 6. Skin Diseases--pathology. W1 CU804L v.39 2010 / WR 218 I16 2010]
RL435.I18 2010
616.5'44--dc22

2010022958

Bibliographic Indices. This publication is listed in bibliographic services, including Current Contents® and Index Medicus.

Disclaimer. The statements, opinions and data contained in this publication are solely those of the individual authors and contributors and not of the publisher and the editor(s). The appearance of advertisements in the book is not a warranty, endorsement, or approval of the products or services advertised or of their effectiveness, quality or safety. The publisher and the editor(s) disclaim responsibility for any injury to persons or property resulting from any ideas, methods, instructions or products referred to in the content or advertisements.

Drug Dosage. The authors and the publisher have exerted every effort to ensure that drug selection and dosage set forth in this text are in accord with current recommendations and practice at the time of publication. However, in view of ongoing research, changes in government regulations, and the constant flow of information relating to drug therapy and drug reactions, the reader is urged to check the package insert for each drug for any change in indications and dosage and for added warnings and precautions. This is particularly important when the recommended agent is a new and/or infrequently employed drug.

www.karger.com
Printed in Switzerland on acid-free and non-aging paper (ISO 9706) by Reinhardt Druck, Basel
ISSN 1421–5721
ISBN 978–3–8055–9394–6
e-ISBN 978–3–8055–9395–3

Contents

Dedication

We would like to dedicate this volume to our ichthyosis patients and their families, from whom – by their courage and positive attitude as well as their generosity of time (and tissue!) – we have learned so much about how people meet the challenges of living continuously with an often debilitating and highly visible skin disease. As we look back over our careers, the advances in understanding these diseases, largely fueled by the molecular biological revolution and the work of many investigators, are truly astonishing. Yet, our ability to treat these disorders has experienced little change. It is our hope that integrating the insights gained from molecular genetics with the dynamics of the epidermal functional response to these disorders will point to new and effective forms of therapy for these disorders.

Preface

The initial impetus for this book, i.e. as an atlas of diagnostic ultrastructure, resulted from a clinical research project of Dr. Anna Bruckner's (Stanford University). As a pediatric dermatology fellow at University of California, San Francisco, from 2004 to 2005 and without prior laboratory experience, Anna's project was to assess whether clinicians, as novices in electron microscopy, could be trained to identify key ultrastructural abnormalities that assist in the diagnosis of different types of ichthyosis. Since Anna readily learned the ultrastructural features of the principal types of ichthyosis [chapter 1, this vol., table 4, pp. 25–26], we realized that by publication of representative images, we could make this structural information more widely available. Yet, because our interests ranged beyond descriptive morphology, this book subsequently evolved from its original scope as an ultrastructural atlas into a text of broader purpose, with substantial additional information on the clinical features, biochemical genetics and the cellular pathogenesis of the (mendelian) monogenic inherited disorders of cornification (MeDOC).

Over the years, we have attempted to unravel the pathogenic mechanisms that lead to the clinical phenotype in many of the MeDOC. While most assessments of disease pathogenesis proceed from the gene to the phenotype ('downstream'), our approach instead looks 'upstream' from the functional abnormalities, which 'drive' the phenotype, towards the responsible gene. Of course, this approach is most productive when the responsible gene is already known. But surprisingly, knowledge of the genetic abnormality often provides few insights into the pathogenesis of the skin phenotype, and instead can mislead the investigator (prominent examples include epidermolytic ichthyosis, loricrin keratoderma and transglutaminase-1-linked lamellar ichthyosis). The appropriateness of this backward-looking approach is evident when one considers the diversity of genetic defects that converge on quite similar phenotypes. These ichthyosiform phenotypes represent the 'best attempt' by the epidermis to sustain a barrier that suffices to allow survival in a xeric, terrestrial environment, i.e. the genetic abnormality partially thwarts this response and an ichthyotic phenotype is the result. Therefore, therapeutic interventions, which are not discussed in this volume, need to be consistent with and, if possible, support this attempt at barrier restoration. Accordingly, while gene replacement therapy still remains a distant dream, knowledge of cellular pathogenic mechanisms could provide immediate opportunities for novel therapies aimed alternatively at disease pathogenesis.

Importantly, the application of ultrastructure to the diagnosis of the ichthyoses requires the utilization of both osmium tetroxide and ruthenium tetroxide (RuO_4) postfixation. Without the utilization of RuO_4, it is not possible to visualize either: (1) the amount of extracellular lipids; (2) the maturation of secreted lamellar body contents, and most importantly, (3) alterations in the structure and organization of the lamellar bilayers themselves. Because successful implementation of RuO_4 postfixation requires substantial training, Ms. Debra Crumrine provides a technical primer in Appendix 1, which we hope will assist laboratories that are attempting to add diagnostic ultrastructure to their morphological armamentarium. Yet, ultrastructural information, though potentially diagnostic, should always be considered provisional, until verified further by biochemical, immunohistochemical or molecular genetic studies. Moreover, this volume is not intended to be comprehensive. There are many disease entities that we have not examined, as well as several that we chose to exclude, most notably the palmar-plantar keratodermas, connexin-related disorders and trichothiodystrophy. Furthermore, we admit that in some instances, the literature cited is incomplete, and, as a result, it may fail to give sufficient credit to those who have made important contributions to the delineation of these entities. A final word of caution: we have no personal experience with the utility of cutaneous ultrastructure for the prenatal diagnosis of the ichthyoses. Because characteristic structural features of children and adults could differ during epidermal development in utero, it should not be assumed that the distinctive structural changes that we describe here for certain MeDOC will necessarily be present in fetal epidermis.

Our work on the pathogenesis and ultrastructural diagnosis of the ichthyoses has been dependent in large part upon the technical and interpretive skills of a master electron microscopy technician, Ms. Debra Crumrine. She has applied, and continues to apply, her highly developed skills to the biopsy material that we receive from all over the world. For Debbie, this project largely represented a labor of love, i.e. a way to help patients with ichthyosis by identifying potentially diagnostic, ultrastructural features of specific disease entities.

This work has been supported by NIH grants AR019098, AR039448(PP), the Medical Research Service of the US Department of Veterans Affairs, the Austrian Science Fund (grants FWF-J1901-MED and FWF-J2112-MED) and the Medical Research Fund of Tirol. Ms. Joan Wakefield, an administrative assistant *extraordinaire*, provided superb editorial assistance not only in the preparation of the text, but she also prepared much of the illustrative materials. We also appreciate the input and comments received from numerous colleagues, including Judith Fischer, Gabriele Richard, Denis Khnykin and Vinzenz Oji, who also contributed an invaluable chapter on disease classification to this volume.

Introduction

Generalized scaling disorders can be of either acquired or inherited etiology. This book focuses solely on generalized, inherited (mendelian) disorders of cornification (DOC or MeDOC), which constitute an ever-enlarging group of monogenic diseases caused by a large number of genes that affect a broad array of cellular functions (table 1). The diagnosis of specific entities within this group largely rests upon recognition of specific clinical features (e.g. the quality and distribution of scales, the neonatal phenotype and the presence or absence of associated cutaneous abnormalities, such as ectropion, keratoderma, centripetal vs. acral involvement, hair shaft anomalies) as well as involvement of other organ systems. With the exception of the characteristic light-microscopic features of epidermolytic ichthyosis (EI; epidermolytic hyperkeratosis, EHK), the droplets positive for oil red O in neutral lipid storage disease and ichthyosis prematurity syndrome (IPS; and the characteristic lamellar inclusions in the corneocyte cytosol in IPS), routine histopathology and ultrastructure do not suffice to allow the correct diagnoses. There are several reasons for this. First, images of the stratum corneum (SC), as viewed by light as well as by routine electron microscopy, are largely artifactual in appearance. For example, because of shrinkage and extraction of extracellular lipids during routine tissue processing, the 'normal basket weave pattern' of the SC in no way reflects the true architecture of this tissue (fig. 1a). If parallel samples instead are viewed as frozen sections (where lipid extraction is avoided) and stained with lipophilic dyes, both the compact, cohesive, organized structure of normal SC, and the localization of lipids to intercellular membrane domains can be appreciated (fig. 1b).

The second reason for the limited utility of light microscopy in the diagnosis of the ichthyoses is perhaps even more important, namely the convergence of a multiplicity of genotypes upon a limited spectrum of clinical phenotypes. This phenotypic convergence can be best understood by consideration of the impact of the mutations on SC function, particularly permeability barrier function, and the homeostatic mechanisms that are activated in an attempt to correct barrier dysfunction – efforts that are at best only partially successful. The metabolic response to barrier failure includes: (1) upregulation of lipid synthesis in nucleated epidermal cell layers and accelerated delivery of more lipids to the SC (the 'make and deliver more lipid!' imperative); (2) epidermal hyperproliferation (the imperative to 'make more cells that in turn will make more lipid'), and (3) inflammation ('protect from invading microorganisms!').

Table 1. Functional classification of the ichthyoses

Category	Disorders
Protease/ antiprotease	Netherton syndrome, Papillon-Lefèvre syndrome
Lipid metabolism	Refsum disease, neutral lipid storage disease with ichthyosis, Sjögren-Larsson syndrome, congenital hemidysplasia with ichthyosiform erythrodermaand limb defects, Conradi-Hünermann-Happle syndrome, recessive X-linked ichthyosis, Gaucher disease
Lipid assembly/ transport	Harlequin ichthyosis, cerebral dysgenesis/neuropathy/ ichthyosis/palmar-plantar keratoderma syndrome, mental retardation/enteropathy/deafness/neuropathy/ ichthyosis/keratoderma syndrome, ichthyosis prematurity syndrome
Keratinopathies	Epidermolytic ichthyosis, superficial epidermolytic ichthyosis
Corneocyte envelope	Loricrin keratoderma, transglutaminase-1-negative lamellar ichthyosis
DNA transcription	Trichothiodystrophy
Cell-to-cell communication	Erythrokeratoderma variabilis, Vohwinkel syndrome (connexins)

Thus, the net consequences of epidermal hyperplasia, hyperkeratosis and inflammation are near-universal features of the ichthyoses. The interplay of this limited array of repair responses confronting the flawed cellular consequences of the specific genotype results in the specific, albeit often overlapping, clinical phenotypes.

Attempts have been made to utilize the higher resolution offered by routine electron microscopy to refine diagnoses of this heterogeneous group of inherited disorders, but an important limitation of routine electron microscopy is that standard techniques do not permit evaluation of either the quantity or the organization of the lipid-enriched, extracellular matrix of the SC. Standard processing of tissue samples for electron microscopy results in the same extraction artifacts that occur during paraffin embedding for light microscopy. Hence, key information about abnormalities in the extracellular compartment of the SC cannot be retrieved. The limited progress to date in delineating the pathogenesis of many of the DOC can be attributed largely to a failure to utilize methods that allow evaluation of dynamic changes in the architecture of affected SC, including not only changes in the organization of the lipid-enriched, extracellular lamellae, but also in corneodesmosome structures within the SC interstices. This problem has been overcome by the development and widespread deployment of ruthenium

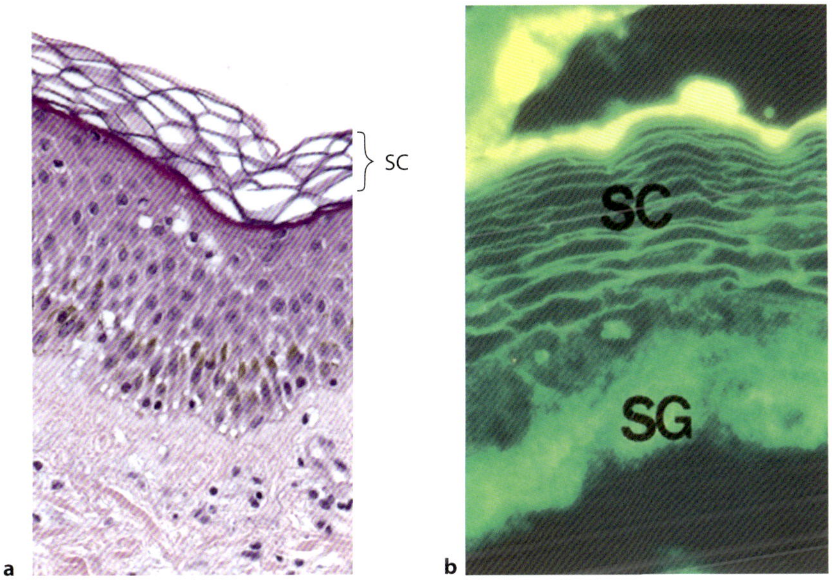

Fig. 1. The SC. **a** 'Normal basket weave' = artifact of lipid extraction during tissue processing. **b** Frozen section stained with hydrophobic dye demonstrating that membrane domains in the SC are neutral and lipid enriched. SG = Stratum granulosum.

tetroxide (RuO_4) postfixation, which resolves key ultrastructural features of the SC extracellular matrix. The failure to include RuO_4-postfixed material in the evaluation of the DOC would be analogous to attempting to diagnose the blistering diseases without the ability to view components of the epidermal basement membrane.

In subsequent sections, we will review the subcellular consequences of many of the genetically characterized DOC, utilizing ultrastructural features captured by the application of a battery of techniques, including (but not limited to) RuO_4 postfixation. In many cases, we show further the impact of these changes for permeability barrier homeostasis. These efforts are still a work in progress, not only because some of the disorders have not yet been characterized at a molecular level, but also because many have not been evaluated using current morphological methods. Nevertheless, many as yet unpublished, potentially diagnostic observations are presented for the first time in this volume, which shed further light on the pathogenesis of several DOC. These ultrastructural studies include Refsum disease, CHILD (congenital hemidysplasia with ichthyosiform erythroderma and limb defects) syndrome, Sjögren-Larsson syndrome, ichthyosis vulgaris, IPS and ichthyosis en confettis.

In Appendix 1, we provide protocols for proper tissue handling, primary fixation, postfixation (OsO_4 and RuO_4), cytochemical and tracer methods, with the intent to spur future efforts to explore the pathogenesis of this fascinating but complex group of disorders. Finally, and most importantly, we believe that this effort is not merely a 'stamp collection' – in understanding how the epidermis fails in these genetic diseases, one can shed new light not only on disease pathogenesis, but also on normal epidermal function.

1.1. Classification of the Ichthyoses (Disorders of Cornification)

The following classification is derived from a consensus paper by Oji et al. [1]. Any references can be obtained from this consensus document.

1.1.1 Recommended Revision of Terminology and Classification of Inherited Ichthyoses

The generic term 'inherited ichthyosis' refers to all MeDOC that are characterized clinically by hyperkeratosis and/or scaling involving most or all of the skin surface. Despite concerns that the term 'ichthyosis', with its reference to fish scales, is potentially pejorative, outmoded and inaccurate, it seems too firmly entrenched in both the literature and in the minds of clinicians to be abandoned. Hence, inherited ichthyoses are regarded as one disease group within the greater group of DOC. To achieve greater clarity, a consensus group gathered recently near Toulouse, France [1], to (re) define some important clinical and dermatological terms that are in common usage. Importantly, the revised classification that emerged includes a specific definition of the term 'autosomal recessive congenital ichthyosis' (ARCI) and major changes in terminology of ichthyoses that are due to keratin mutations.

1.1.2 General Framework for the Revised Classification Scheme

At present, molecular diagnosis is not available for all forms of ichthyosis, and access to genetic diagnostics can be impeded by geographic availability or by cost-related concerns. Similarly, ultrastructural techniques are not in common clinical use by pathologists and are not widely available to clinicians. Other laboratory techniques, including light microscopy, can narrow the differential diagnosis in only a few cases, but decisions regarding further testing, i.e. molecular diagnostics, rest upon rigorous, initial clinical evaluations. Therefore, a clinically based classification was retained, in which the DOC are referenced with their causative gene(s). Two principal groups are recognized: nonsyndromic and syndromic forms (fig. 2). This algorithm is in the tradition of previous concepts and is based upon whether the phenotype is only expressed in the skin (prototypes: lamellar ichthyosis, LI, and EI) versus whether skin manifestations are part of a wider disease expression with involvement of multiple organs. For purposes of this classification, recessive X-linked ichthyosis (RXLI) is otherwise considered nonsyndromic and is regarded as syndromic only when it is

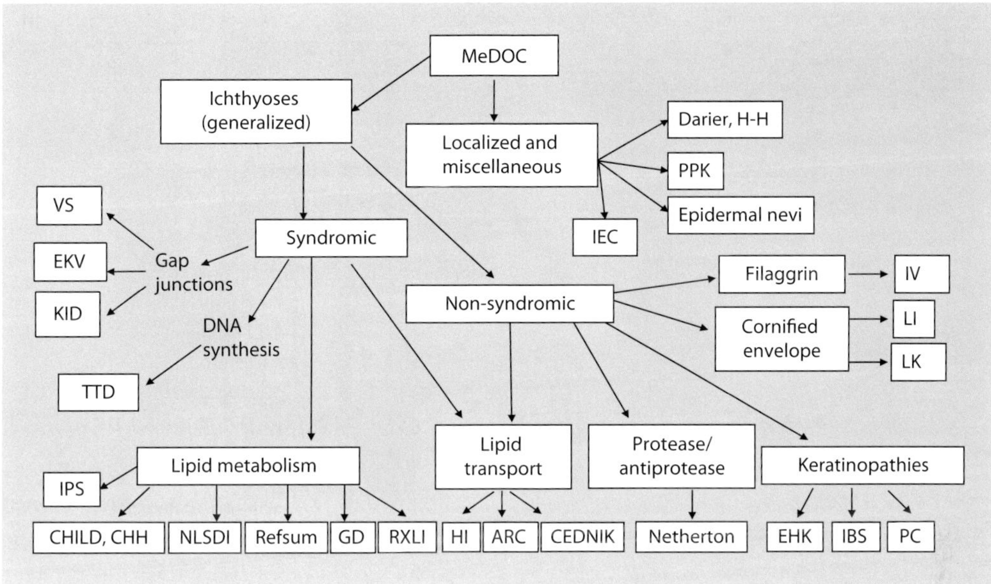

Fig. 2. Overview of the MeDOC. ARC = Arthrogryposis/renal dysfunction/cholestasis syndrome; CEDNIK = cerebral dysgenesis, neuropathy, ichthyosis and palmar-plantar keratoderma; CHH = Conradi-Hünermann-Happle syndrome; EKV = erythrokeratoderma variabilis; GD = Gaucher disease; H-H = Hailey-Hailey disease; HI = harlequin ichthyosis; IBS = ichthyosis bullosa of Siemens (epidermolysis bullosa simplex); IEC = ichthyosis en confettis; IV = ichthyosis vulgaris; KID = keratitis/ichthyosis/deafness syndrome; LI = lamellar ichthyosis; LK = loricrin keratoderma; NLSDI = neutral lipid storage disease with ichthyosis (Chanarin-Dorfman syndrome); PC = pachyonychia congenita; PPK = palmar-plantar keratoderma; RXLI = recessive X-linked ichthyosis; TTD = trichothiodystrophy; VS = Vohwinkel syndrome.

accompanied by associated extracutaneous manifestations, such as undescended testes. To facilitate identification of the syndromic ichthyoses, subheadings are included that point to the most prominent, associated disorders (table 2).

In the past, many authorities have emphasized the distinction between congenital ichthyoses versus ichthyoses of delayed onset, such as ichthyosis vulgaris and RXLI. Yet, even in these delayed-onset disorders, early subtle skin changes may be overlooked, e. g. RXLI may present shortly after birth with fine superficial scaling, which can fade initially but then reappear as a clear ichthyosis later in life. Thus, because of the high variability of initial disease presentation, the age of onset has not been chosen as major criterion of classification.

1.1.3 Classification of Autosomal Recessive Congenital Ichthyoses

The acronym ARCI was proposed as an umbrella term for the former LI/congenital ichthyosiform erythroderma (CIE) spectrum patients. Harlequin ichthyosis (HI) is

Table 2. Syndromic forms of inherited ichthyosis

Disease	Mode of inheritance	Gene(s)
X-linked syndromes		
Recessive X-linked ichthyosis	X-linked recessive	*STS* (and others[1])
Ichthyosis follicularis/alopecia/photophobia syndrome	X-linked recessive	*MBTPS2*
Conradi-Hünermann-Happle syndrome	X-linked dominant	*EBP (CDPX2)*[2]
Autosomal ichthyosis syndromes		
+ prominent hair abnormalities		
Netherton syndrome	autosomal recessive	*SPINK5*
Ichthyosis/hypotrichosis syndrome	autosomal recessive	*ST14*[3]
Ichthyosis/hypotrichosis/sclerosing cholangitis syndrome	autosomal recessive	*CLDN1*[4]
Trichothiodystrophy (congenital)	autosomal recessive	*ERCC2/XPD* *ERCC3/XPB* *GTF2H5/TTDA*
Trichothiodystrophy (noncongenital)	autosomal recessive	*C7Orf11/TTDN1*
+ prominent neurological involvement		
Sjögren-Larsson syndrome	autosomal recessive	*ALDH3A2*
Refsum syndrome (HMSN4)	autosomal recessive	*PHYH/PEX7*
Mental retardation/enteropathy/deafness/ neuropathy/ichthyosis/keratoderma syndrome	autosomal recessive	*AP1S1*
+ progressive, fatal course		
Gaucher disease type 2	autosomal recessive	*GBA*
Multiple sulfatase deficiency	autosomal recessive	*SUMF1*
Cerebral dysgenesis/neuropathy/ichthyosis/ palmoplantar keratoderma sydrome	autosomal recessive	*SNAP29*
Arthrogryposis/renal dysfunction/cholestasis syndrome	autosomal recessive	*VPS33B*
+ other signs		
Keratitis/ichthyosis/deafness syndrome	autosomal dominant	*GJB2 (GJB6)*
Neutral lipid storage disease with ichthyosis	autosomal recessive	*ABHD5*
Ichthyosis prematurity syndrome	autosomal recessive	*SLC27A4*

[1] In the context of a contiguous gene syndrome.
[2] Chondrodysplasia punctata type 2; hereditary motor and sensory neuropathy type 4 (HMSN4).
[3] Clinical variant: congenital ichthyosis, follicular atrophoderma, hypotrichosis and hypohidrosis syndrome.
[4] Also known as neonatal ichthyosis/sclerosing cholangitis syndrome.

included, because functional null mutations in the *ABCA12* gene cause the disease, whereas missense mutations in the same gene may be associated with a milder phenotype that shows a collodion membrane at birth and subsequently develops into an LI or CIE phenotype, often with palmar-plantar keratoderma. Infants with null mutations, who survive the perinatal period, also go on later to express a severe, scaling erythroderma, further underscoring the rationale for inclusion of HI within the ARCI group.

One difficulty of the ARCI classification is the limited information that is available about genotype-phenotype correlations within the LI/CIE spectrum. Mutations in 6 genes have been described in non-HI ARCI to date, including *TGM1*, the gene encoding transglutaminase 1 (TGM-1), the genes *ABCA12*, *NIPAL4* (also known as ichthyin), *CYP4F22* and the lipoxygenase genes *ALOX12B* and *ALOXE3*. But about one quarter of ARCI cases do not exhibit mutations in any of the known ARCI genes, implying that further loci must exist, of which 2 loci on chromosome 12p11.2–q13 are candidates. A preliminary clinicogenetic correlation is provided here, based upon both the recent literature and on discussions at the consensus conference [1].

LI is characterized by coarse and brown/dark scales, and affected individuals are often born with a collodion membrane and pronounced ectropion [see chapter 4, this vol., pp. 98–127, for further clinical details]. CIE is characterized by fine, white scaling with varying degrees of erythema. CIE patients who are born with a collodion membrane (usually less severe than in LI), then transit to generalized fine scaling and pronounced erythroderma. Clinical phenotypes can change over time and in response to treatment, e.g. retinoid-treated LI can turn into an erythrodermic ichthyosis with fine scales, as in CIE. In a recent North American study of 104 patients with non-HI ARCI, mutations in *TGM1* were significantly associated with collodion membrane, ectropion, plate-like scales and alopecia. Patients with at least 1 truncation mutation of *TGM1* were more likely to display severe hypohidrosis and overheating than do patients with only *TGM1* missense mutations.

Other minor ARCI variants/subtypes can be distinguished clinically: bathing suit ichthyosis has been attributed to particular *TGM1* mutations that render the enzyme sensitive to ambient temperature. The self-resolving collodion baby, representing approximately 10% of all ARCI cases, has so far been associated with *TGM1*, *ALOXE3* or *ALOX12B* mutations. The recently described acral self-resolving collodion baby, i.e. with collodion membranes at birth that are strictly localized to the extremities and then heal, can also be due to *TGM1* mutations.

1.1.4 Classification of the Keratinopathic Ichthyoses

The term 'EI' (tables 2 and 3) [chapter 4, this vol., pp. 98–127] derives from the characteristic light-microscopic descriptive term 'EHK' for the constellation of intracellular vacuolization, clumping of tonofilaments and formation of small intraepidermal

Table 3. Nonsyndromic forms of ichthyosis (primary)

Disease	Mode of inheritance	Gene(s)
Common ichthyoses		
Ichthyosis vulgaris	autosomal semidominant	*FLG*
Recessive X-linked ichthyosis (most)	X-linked recessive	*STS*
Autosomal recessive congenital ichthyosis		
Major types		
Harlequin ichthyosis	autosomal recessive	*ABCA12*
Lamellar ichthyosis[1]	autosomal recessive	*TGM1/NIPAL4*[2]*/ ALOX12B/ABCA12* (loci on 12p11.2–q13)
Congenital ichthyosiform erythroderma	autosomal recessive	*ALOXE3/ALOX12B/ ABCA12/CYP4F22/ NIPAL4*[2]*/TGM1* (loci on 12p11.2–q13)
Minor variants		
Self-resolving collodion baby	autosomal recessive	*TGM1/ALOX12B*
Acral self-resolving collodion baby	autosomal recessive	*TGM1*
Bathing suit ichthyosis	autosomal recessive	*TGM1*
Keratinopathic ichthyosis		
Major types		
Epidermolytic ichthyosis[3]	autosomal dominant	*K1/K10*
Superficial epidermolytic ichthyosis	autosomal dominant	*K2*
Minor variants		
Annular epidermolytic ichthyosis	autosomal dominant	*K1/K10*
Ichthyosis Curth-Macklin	autosomal dominant	*K1*
Autosomal recessive epidermolytic ichthyosis	autosomal recessive	*K10*
Epidermolytic nevi[4]	somatic mutations	*K1/K10*

Table 3. Continued

Disease	Mode of inheritance	Gene(s)
Other forms		
Loricrin keratoderma	autosomal dominant	*LOR*
Erythrokeratoderma variabilis[5]	autosomal dominant	*GJB3/GJB4*
Peeling skin syndrome	autosomal recessive	TGM5/? SPINK5 (most unknown)
Congenital reticular ichthyosiform erythroderma	autosomal dominant(?) (isolated cases)	locus unknown
Keratosis linearis/ichthyosis congenita/keratoderma	autosomal recessive	13q

[1] A few cases of autosomal dominant lamellar ichthyosis have been described (loci unknown).
[2] Also known as ichthyin gene.
[3] *K1* mutations are often associated with palmoplantar involvement.
[4] May indicate a gonadal mosaicism, which can cause generalized EI in offspring.
[5] Whether progressive symmetric erythrokeratoderma comprises a distinct MeDOC form is debatable.

blisters. The term 'EHK' has been used (by some) as synonymous for 'bullous ichthyosis', 'ichthyosis exfoliativa', 'bullous CIE (of Brocq)' and 'ichthyosis bullosa of Siemens'. Notably, the light-microscopic features of EHK may not be observed in all instances of the keratinopathic ichthyoses, but they can be detected readily on electron microscopy [chapter 4, this vol., pp. 98–127]. To replace this long list of terms, the consensus group proposed a new umbrella term, keratinopathic ichthyosis, that encompasses all of these entities (table 3). The new term EI now applies to clinical disorders known to be due to keratin 1 *(K1)* or *K10* mutations, to avoid the use of a histopathological term (EHK), which should henceforth be used exclusively as a histopathological descriptor. The novel disease term 'superficial EI' is now proposed for the related, well-defined entity, formerly termed 'ichthyosis bullosa of Siemens', which shows a more superficial pattern of epidermolysis than EI and is caused by mutations in keratin 2, rather than keratins 1 or 10.

Clinically, the keratinopathic ichthyoses show a broad spectrum of skin manifestations and severity. While widespread skin blistering is characteristic of neonates with EI, the blistering phenotype evolves into a hyperkeratotic (barrier-driven) phenotype ('phenotypic shift'), which is due to impaired lamellar body secretion, rather than corneocyte fragility [chapter 4, this vol., pp. 98–127]. Superficial EI has a milder phenotype and can be distinguished from EI by its lack of erythroderma and a characteristic 'molting' phenomenon. In all EI, light microscopy and standard electron microscopy reveal cytolysis that correlates with the restricted expression of keratin 2 in the stratum granulosum and upper stratum spinosum. Annular EI, which is due to *K1* or *K10* mutations, is now classified as a clinical variant of EI. Different features, including distribution, erythema or blistering, distinguish 6 clinical subgroups of EI, but the most distinctive characteristic is the involvement of palms and soles (PS 1–3 vs. NPS 1–3). Palmar-plantar keratoderma is usually predictive of a *K1* mutation, perhaps because keratin 9, which is expressed in palm and sole epidermis, may compensate for the keratin 10 defect, while keratin 1 is the only type 2 keratin expressed in palmar-plantar epidermis. Nonetheless, palmar-plantar keratoderma has been reported with *K10* mutations as well.

As with pachyonychia congenita and the epidermolysis bullosa simplex group, the vast majority of the keratinopathic ichthyosis cases result from autosomal dominant mutations. These mutations result in the expression of an abnormal keratin protein that interferes with the formation (assembly) and/or function of keratin intermediate filaments, often leading to keratin intermediate filament aggregation and cytolysis, which in turn interfere with lamellar body secretion [chapter 4, this vol., pp. 98–127]. However, *K10* nonsense mutations have been observed that do not lead to the usual 'dominant negative effect' and cause an autosomal recessive form of keratinopathic ichthyosis. Therefore, autosomal recessive EI is listed as new and discrete keratinopathic ichthyosis. Ichthyosis Curth-Macklin represents a very rare form of keratinopathic ichthyosis that shows a unique ultrastructure; the adjective 'hystrix' has been omitted but the eponym Curth-Macklin retained. Hystrix-like skin changes can be observed in other ichthyoses, e.g. keratitis/ichthyosis/deafness (KID) syndrome, or in particular types of epidermal nevi. Finally and importantly, some epidermolytic nevi, i.e. those that exhibit the histopathology of EHK, indicate a somatic type 1 mosaicism for mutations in *K1* or *K10*, which, if also gonadal, can result in generalized EI in the patient's offspring. Because recognition of this risk is important for genetic counseling, epidermolytic nevi are included here in the classification of keratinopathic ichthyosis.

1.1.5 Other Diseases That Fall within the Umbrella of Inherited Ichthyoses

Additional ichthyoses described in the literature include: ichthyosis follicularis/atrichia/photophobia syndrome, multiple sulfatase deficiency, congenital reticular ichthyosiform erythroderma also referred to as ichthyosis variegata and ichthyosis en confettis [chapter 5, this vol., pp. 128–132]. IPS has to be distinguished from self-resolving collodion babies, because, while in both diseases the skin improves dramatically soon after birth, IPS represents a distinct genetic disorder due to deficiency of a fatty acid transporter [chapter 2, this vol., pp. 30–88]. Recent studies on genotype-phenotype correlation distinguish the heterogeneous group of trichothiodystrophies as either those associated with ichthyosis of delayed onset or those preceded by a collodion membrane phenotype. Diseases relatively new to the list of ichthyoses include [chapter 2, this vol., pp. 30–88]: (1) cerebral dysgenesis/neuropathy/ichthyosis/palmar-plantar keratoderma (CEDNIK) syndrome; (2) arthrogryposis/renal dysfunction/cholestasis syndrome; (3) mental retardation/enteropathy/deafness/neuropathy/ichthyosis/keratoderma (MEDNIK) syndrome; (4) ichthyosis/hypotrichosis/sclerosing cholangitis syndrome; (5) ichthyosis hypotrichosis syndrome and its allelic variant congenital ichthyosis/follicular atrophoderma/hypotrichosis/hypohidrosis syndrome, as well as (6) keratosis linearis/ichthyosis/congenital sclerosing keratoderma.

Erythrokeratoderma variabilis (EKV), which is characterized by migratory erythematous patches with more fixed, symmetrical hyperkeratotic plaques, often with palmar-plantar involvement, is genetically heterogeneous and caused by mutations in *GJB3*, which encodes the gap junction protein connexin 31, or *GJB4* coding for connexin 30.3. EKV may be localized or generalized. Another connexin disorder, KID syndrome, is identical to ichthyosis hystrix, type Rheydt, or hystrix-like ichthyosis/deafness syndrome. KID syndrome is due to heterozygous mutations in *GJB2* (connexin 26). Patients with a congenital presentation usually have generalized skin involvement. In some cases, KID syndrome, like Clouston syndrome, is caused by mutations in *GJB6* (connexin 30). Whether progressive symmetric erythrokeratoderma, which displays considerable clinical overlap with EKV, comprises a distinct disease entity is unclear at present. Although it is generally considered a distinct entity, patients from 2 progressive symmetric erythrokeratoderma families displayed the same *GJB4* mutation as in others with EKV.

One could argue that Netherton syndrome (NS) should not be classified with the ichthyoses, since it is characterized by premature desquamation and a thinner, rather than a thicker SC [chapter 3, this vol., pp. 89–97]. However, scaling is a prominent clinical feature, often resembling a CIE phenotype. Unlike NS, the peeling skin syndrome does not show hair anomalies and shows different immunochemical features; nonetheless, some cases have demonstrated *TG5* or *SPINK5* mutations [chapter 3, this vol., pp. 89–97]. Like NS, peeling skin syndrome may also be accompanied by an atopic diathesis.

A certain number of MeDOC forms can be regarded as phenotypically and/or etiologically related to ichthyosis, or they should be considered in their differential diagnosis. Examples include palmar-plantar keratoderma, which sometimes shows nonacral involvement, as in Vohwinkel syndrome, caused by a dominant *GJB2* mutation (connexin 26), mal de Meleda, caused by recessive *SLURP1* mutations, and Papillon-Lefèvre syndrome, caused by recessive *CTSC* mutations encoding cathepsin C. Lethal restrictive dermopathy is in the differential diagnosis of HI (and severe collodion babies) and is associated with intrauterine growth retardation, congenital contractures, tight skin and ectropion, but not hyperkeratosis or scaling. Another perinatal lethal syndrome, the Neu-Laxova syndrome, should be considered in neonates with ichthyosis and multiple anomalies. Here, the skin is tight and translucent, as in restrictive dermopathy, exhibiting an abnormal facies with exophthalmos, marked intrauterine growth retardation, limb deformities and CNS anomalies. CHILD syndrome that is strictly limited to one side of the body does not fulfill the criterion of a *generalized* cornification disorder. CHILD and Conradi-Hünermann-Happle (CDPX2) syndromes both are caused by defects in the distal cholesterol biosynthetic pathway due to X-linked dominant mutations in the *EBP* (CDPX2) and *NSDHL* gene (CHILD), respectively [chapter 2, this vol., pp. 30–88]. CDPX2 may present with severe CIE or collodion membrane. Finally, Darier disease and Hailey-Hailey disease are common autosomal dominant genodermatoses often referred to as 'acantholytic disorders.' They represent MeDOC, in which the formation and/or stability of the keratinocytic desmosomal adhesion is altered by a defect of a sarco(endo)plasmic reticulum Ca^{2+}-ATPase pump (Darier: *ATP2A2* gene) or a secretory Ca^{2+}/Mn^{2+}-ATPase pump of the Golgi apparatus (Hailey-Hailey: *ATP2C1* gene). The typical lesions of Darier disease, which usually begin in adolescence, are tiny keratotic papules, with a firmly adherent keratin cap, most often restricted to a seborrheic distribution, and the scalp and extremities. A detailed overview of disease onset, initial clinical presentation, disease course, cutaneous and extracutaneous findings for these additional entities is given in the consensus report [1]. Finally, a stepwise approach for the workup of a new patient with ichthyosis is provided in figure 3.

1.2. Synopsis of Normal Stratum Corneum Structure and Function

The SC comprises a unique, 2-compartment system of protein-enriched corneocytes, embedded in a lipid-enriched extracellular matrix, analogized to a brick wall [2, 3] (fig. 4). The lipids in normal SC are composed of relatively hydrophobic species, organized into repeating arrays of broad lamellar membranes that completely engorge the extracellular spaces (fig. 5). Consequently, these membranes provide a continuous lamellar phase that spans multiple cell layers, completely enveloping the corneocytes (fig. 4, 5). This organized lipid shield forms the permeability barrier to the outward movement of water through the SC, while simultaneously excluding ingress of noxious chemicals, allergens and microbial pathogens. In normal epidermis, the permeability barrier is first generated at the interface between the stratum granulosum and SC, where the secreted contents of epidermal lamellar bodies disperse and reorganize to form the lamellar membrane structures [4]. Lamellar bodies themselves are multifunctional, lysosome-like organelles that secrete a broad variety of lipid hydrolases, proteases/antiproteases, antimicrobial peptides, apolipoproteins and other proteins, in addition to lipids, into the extracellular spaces [5]. The movement of these organelles to the cell periphery in anticipation of secretion is dependent upon a set of colocalized motor and nonmotor proteins, such as Rab7 and 11, CLIP-170, Cdc42 and Arf [5, 6]. The importance of these proteins is shown by CEDNIK, MEDNIK and

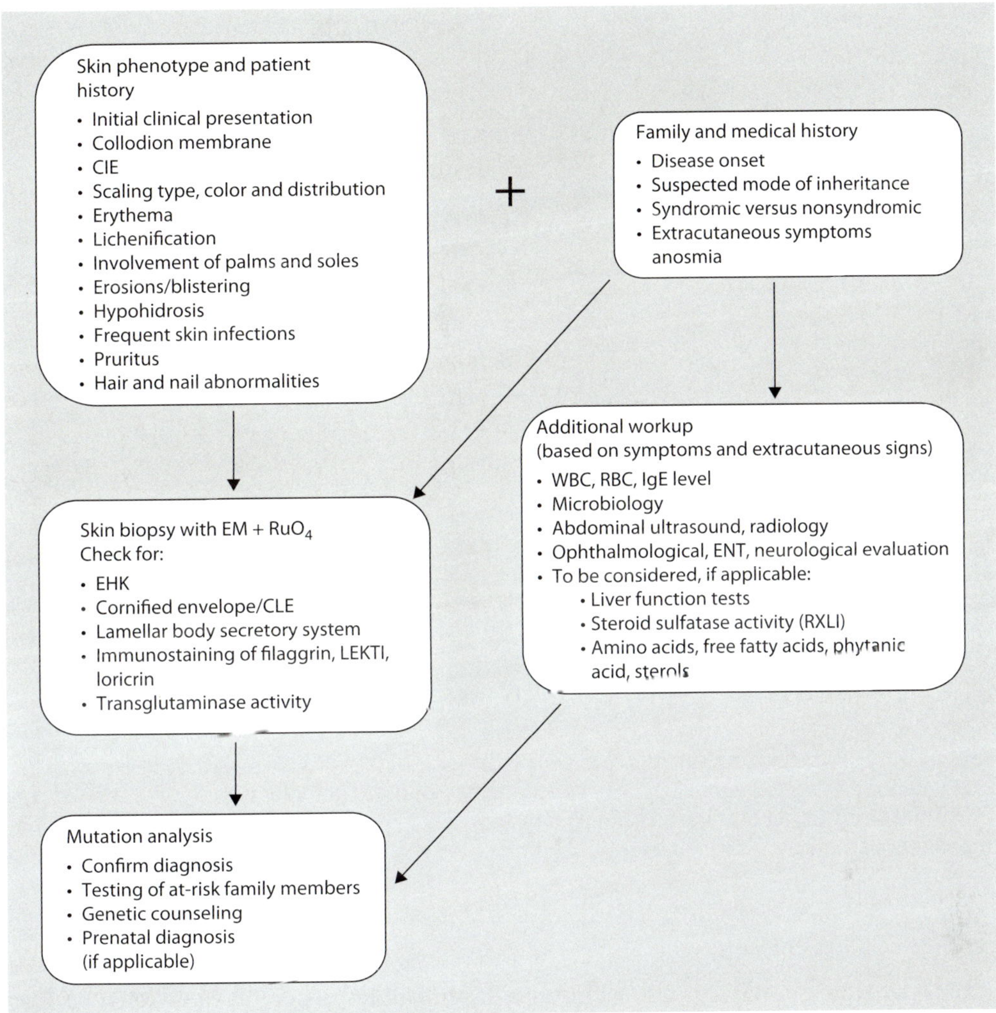

Fig. 3. Evaluation and workup of MeDOC patients (modified from Oji et al. [1]). EM = Electron microscopy; CLE = corneocyte lipid envelope; LEKTI = lymphoepithelial Kazal-type inhibitor.

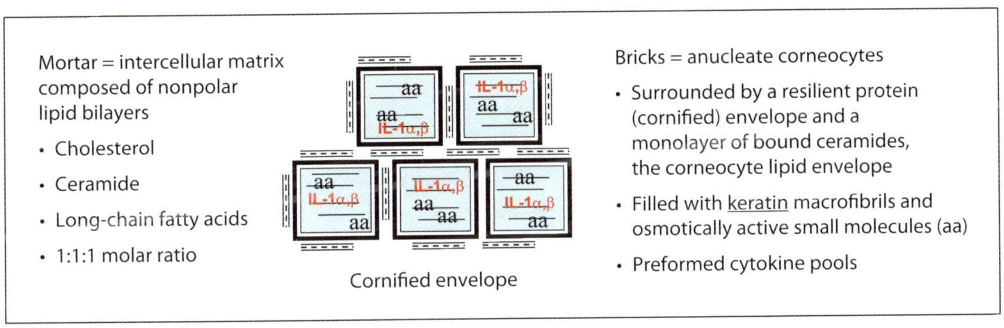

Fig. 4. SC 'bricks-and-mortar' analogy.

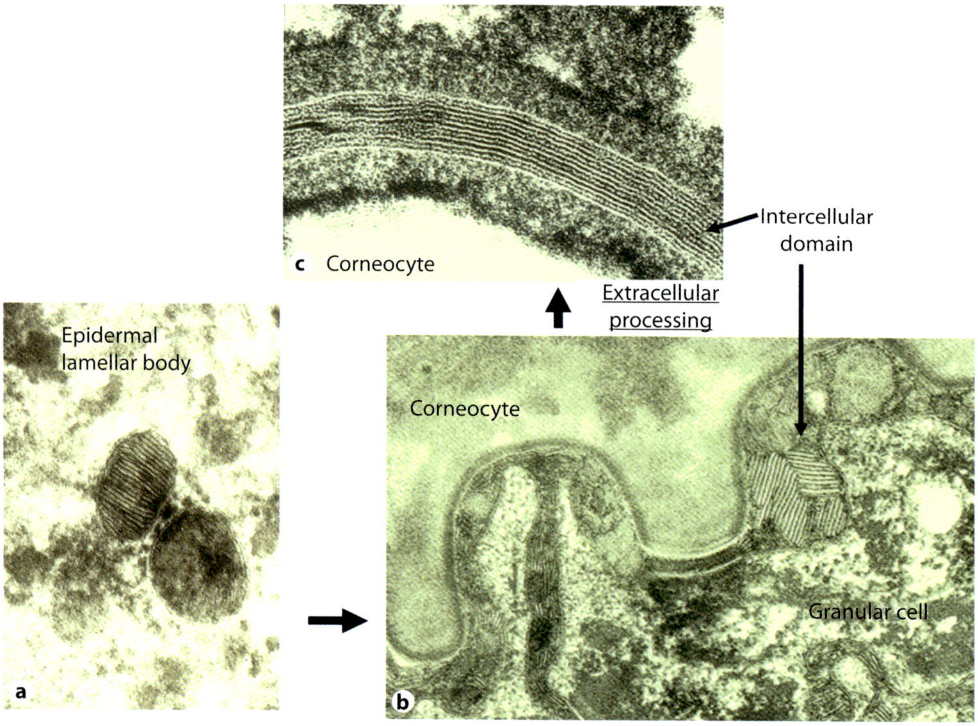

Fig. 5. Normal Lamellar Body Secretory System. **a** Lamellar bodies display replete lamellar contents. **b** Lamellar bodies secrete lamellar contents at interface of outer granular cells and lowermost corneocytes. **c** Secreted lamellar body contents transform into arrays of elongated lamellar bilayers that completely fill the intercellular spaces.

arthrogryposis/renal dysfunction/cholestasis syndromes, where in each instance, loss of one of these proteins results in a severe, syndromic form of ichthyosis.

But the corneocyte 'bricks' are also critical contributors to the permeability barrier, through at least 2 mechanisms. First, corneocytes serve as a critical *scaffold*, required for the organization of the extracellular lipid matrix into its characteristic lamellar pattern, as demonstrated in TGM-1-negative LI, where secretion is normal, but membrane arrays are foreshortened and are only found in regions where the cornified envelope is relatively preserved [7]. Second, the vertical organization of the corneocytes through the generation of multiple, overlapping layers of interdigitating cells (fig. 1b) results in the extracellular matrix forming an elongated and tortuous pathway that further impedes the egress of water [8]. In addition to contributing a key scaffold for the permeability barrier, corneocytes serve several other critical functions. These include *mechanical resilience*, *SC hydration*, *UVB filtration* and additional *pH-dependent* functions related to the humidity-dependent hydrolysis of filaggrin into amino acids and their deiminated products (fig. 4). In addition, they contain a storage pool of preforms of cytokines, IL-1α/β, poised to initiate the cytokine proinflammatory cascade (fig. 4). Finally, the corneocyte envelope is surrounded by a monolayer of covalently bound ω-OH ceramides and ω-OH fatty acids, the corneocyte lipid envelope, which not only links the corneocytes to the extracellular matrix, but also plays key roles in intercorneocyte cohesion and SC hydration, functioning as a semipermeable membrane that seals osmotically active molecules within the corneocyte, while still allowing transmembrane passage of water [9].

Experimental perturbations of the permeability barrier (e.g. through solvent extraction or tape strippings) stimulate a series of homeostatic responses aimed at restoring function [10, 11]. In the first wave of responses, occurring within minutes after acute barrier disruption, loss of the high calcium milieu bathing the outer stratum granulosum signals the secretion of preformed lamellar bodies from the outermost cells of the stratum granulosum (imperative: 'deliver critical lipids quickly!'). In the second phase, occurring within hours, and signaled in part by the release of preformed IL-1α/β from SC stores (fig. 4), epidermal lipid synthesis increases (imperative: 'make more lipid!'). In the third phase, beginning by 16 h, and also in response to cytokine signaling, epidermal DNA synthesis increases (imperative: 'make more cells!' – which then will 'make more lipid'). In normal human epidermis, these responses result in repair of the permeability barrier within about 3 days [12]. In the DOC, a variety of unrelated mutations provoke a barrier defect that cannot be corrected by these homeostatic responses. Because normal function cannot be restored, these repair efforts (hypermetabolism, hyperplasia) do not terminate. Hence, the ichthyoses are invariably associated with epidermal hyperplasia, hyperkeratosis, inflammation and sustained barrier dysfunction.

1.3. Historical Pathogenic Concepts

The DOC comprise a large group of heritable scaling disorders of diverse etiology [13–16]. To date, mutations in more than 30 genes that encode a wide spectrum of proteins are associated with ichthyotic phenotypes, including: (i) enzymes of lipid metabolism; (ii) enzymes of peptide cross-linking; (iii) proteases and their inhibitors; (iv) epidermal structural proteins; (v) proteins of vesicle formation and transport proteins engaged in cell-to-cell communication, and finally (vi) DNA repair enzymes (tables 1–3). Nevertheless, abnormalities in any of these diverse processes result in a rather stereotypic (i.e. limited) epidermal response, characterized by epidermal hyperplasia leading to the formation of excess SC, and abnormal desquamation, with visible accumulation of scaling and/or coarsening of the skin surface with accentuation of the epidermal ridges (hyperkeratosis), with or without underlying erythema – the clinical hallmarks of all the ichthyoses [for reviews, see 17–21].

As knowledge began to accumulate about these disorders, various classification systems were proposed, which then evolved over time into other mechanistic schemes. In the 1960s, Frost et al. [22] offered a classification based upon epidermal kinetics, in which disorders were designated as either *retention* hyperkeratoses (delayed

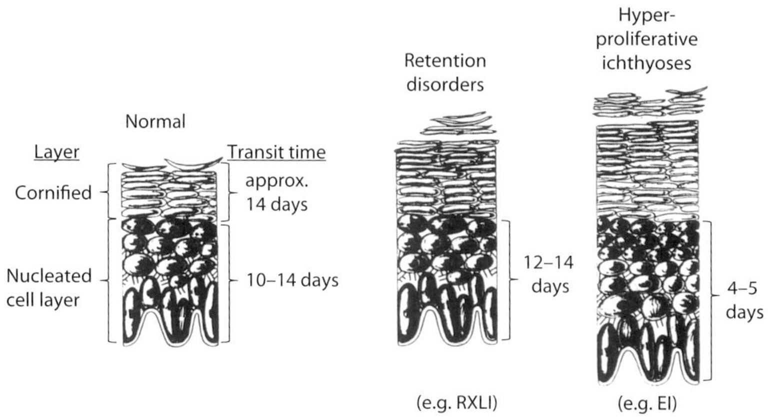

Fig. 6. Classification of DOC based upon epidermal kinetics (modified from Frost et al. [22]).

desquamation with normal rates of epidermal renewal, as in RXLI) or *hyperproliferative* ichthyoses (e.g. EI; fig. 6).

In the 1980s, Williams and Elias [23] and Williams [24] advanced a morphological classification of the DOC as disorders that either affect the extracellular lipids ('mortar') or those that affect structural or enzymatic proteins of the corneocyte ('bricks').

This approach yielded two key insights: (1) that disorders of lipid metabolism alone can alter the extracellular matrix sufficiently to provoke ichthyotic disorders and (2) that extracellular lipids contribute to the cohesive properties of normal SC. Yet, this approach failed to illuminate the functional interdependence of the 'bricks' and 'mortar' compartments. Moreover, it did not incorporate pathogenic consequences resulting from repair responses that are aimed at restoring altered barrier function either, i.e. barrier failure causes epidermal hyperplasia and cytokine signaling of inflammation (see below).

1.4. Function-Driven Pathogenesis of the Ichthyoses

The complex structural and functional interdependence of the cytosolic and extracellular matrix constituents of the SC renders a 'bricks-and-mortar' scheme overly simplistic (fig. 7). For example, the extracellular matrix contains not only lamellar-body-derived lipids, but also corneodesmosome components such as corneodesmosin, which mediate intercorneocyte cohesion, as well as a variety of enzymes that modulate SC functions (fig. 8). Finally, lamellar bodies also deliver at least 2 key antimicrobial peptides, the human cathelicidin carboxyterminal fragment LL-37 and human β-defensin 2 [26, 27]. Accordingly, disorders that result in either decreased

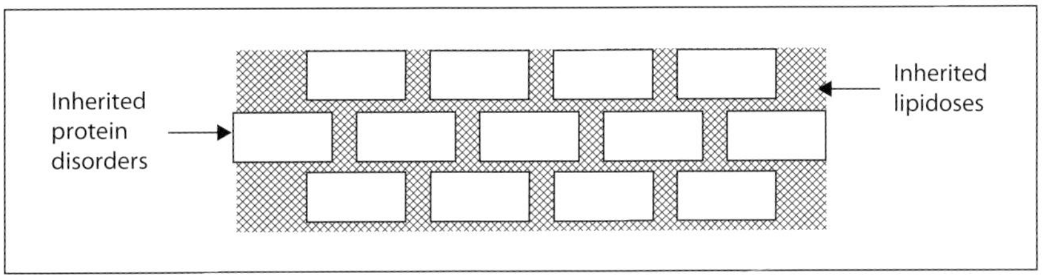

Fig. 7. Classification of ichthyoses as protein (brick) or lipid (mortar) disorders (modified from Williams and Elias [23]).

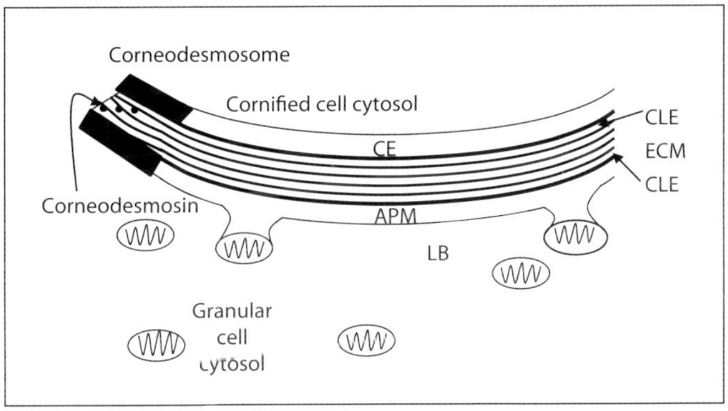

Fig. 8. SC membrane domains (modified from Schmuth et al. [27]). LB = Lamellar body, containing: cholesterol esters, triglycerides, free fatty acids, proteases/antiproteases, antimicrobial peptides, corneodesmosin; ECM = extracellular matrix, containing: lamellar bilayers, antimicrobial peptides, serine/cysteine/aspartate, proteases, protease inhibitors; CLE = cornified lipid envelope, containing: ω-hydroxyceramides/ω-OH free fatty acids; CE = cornified envelope, containing: TGM-1, involucrin, loricrin, keratin, profilaggrin/filaggrin, apical plasma membrane (APM).

delivery or accelerated destruction of secreted lamellar body contents are associated with an increased risk of infection (e.g. EI, HI, NS; fig. 7).

Moreover, it is apparent from studies of inherited defects of both corneocyte envelope proteins (TGM-1-negative LI and loricrin keratoderma) and of defects in the keratin cytoskeleton (e.g. EI) that a competent SC extracellular matrix requires a structurally competent corneocyte. Thus, all of the ichthyoses that are attributable to corneocyte protein abnormalities provoke a secondary defect in the extracellular matrix, which allows accelerated transcutaneous water movement purely via the extracellular pathway [25]. Abnormal permeability barrier function, in turn, drives compensatory manifestations, including epidermal hyperplasia, leading to hyperkeratosis and visible scaling (see below).

As further insights have been gained into the relationships between SC structure and epidermal permeability barrier function [28], it became possible to integrate the epidermal kinetic model with the 'bricks-and-mortar' model. This new, function-driven model provides a framework for understanding how such a broad and disparate group of genetic abnormalities can provoke often similar ichthyotic phenotypes. A key concept of the function-driven model is the recognition that epidermal permeability barrier function is abnormal to a varying extent in most, if not all, of these disorders. While still a work in progress, this function-driven model of pathogenesis provides a rational framework for understanding the convergent clinical phenotypes of this genetically diverse group of genetic disorders. Moreover, this model integrates well with prior histometric and morphological ('bricks-and-mortar') models of the DOC, and importantly, it provides (i) insights into mechanisms of disease, (ii) potential prognostic indicators, and finally (iii) it can guide the development of rational therapeutic approaches [29, 30]. This book provides disease-by-disease information on the subcellular pathogenesis of the ichthyoses, using this function-driven concept.

1.5. Permeability Barrier Dysfunction as the 'Driver' of Disease Expression

To reiterate, regardless of the underlying genetic abnormality, all of the DOC studied to date have demonstrated a permeability barrier abnormality [15, 17, 31–33]. Since permeability barrier requirements generally 'drive' metabolic responses in the underlying epidermis (see above), the clinical phenotypes in the DOC almost certainly reflect a 'best effort' attempt by the epidermis to normalize permeability barrier function [15]. Notably, these metabolic responses to a flawed barrier, though only partially successful in the DOC, nevertheless suffice to allow survival in a dry, terrestrial environment. Even in HI, where few, if any, lipids are delivered to the SC interstices [34–36], the epidermis compensates with an intense, hyperplastic response (increased cell proliferation in response to a highly defective barrier) that generates multiple layers of corneocytes (again, the 'make more cells' imperative) [15] (see above). Furthermore, in inherited disorders that affect the structural proteins of the corneocyte 'bricks', permeability barrier abnormalities result from downstream alterations in the extracellular matrix (see above), albeit by divergent mechanisms. For example, TGM-1-negative LI and loricrin keratoderma represent disorders in which the key cross-linking enzyme and its principal substrate (loricrin), involved in the formation of the corneocyte envelope, are affected (fig. 9).

In both of these disorders, the corneocyte envelope is attenuated, resulting in a defective corneocyte scaffold and leading in turn to fragmented and foreshortened lamellar membranes [7, 37]. It is these altered membranes that result in an impaired barrier, with leakage of water via the extracellular pathway, as can be demonstrated using the water-soluble tracer lanthanum to follow the movement of water through the SC. Pertinently, the cohydroxyceramide-enriched corneocyte lipid envelope, which forms a continuous monolayer around the corneocyte, is normal in both of

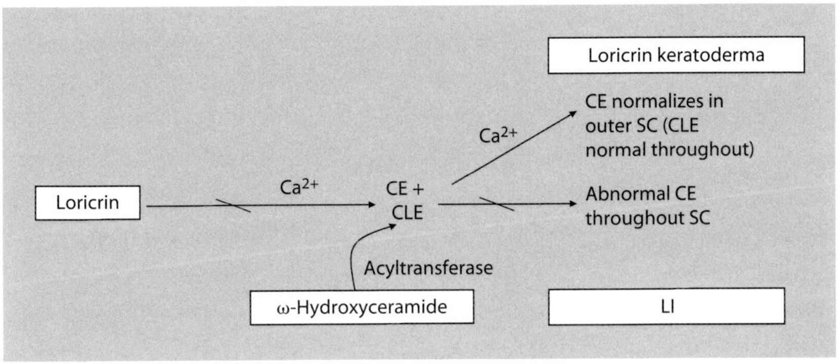

Fig. 9. Scaffold abnormalities in LI and loricrin keratoderma. CE = Corneocyte envelope; CLE = corneocyte lipid envelope.

these disorders, suggesting other non-scaffold-related functions for this structure. Thus, it is the link between a defective corneocyte envelope and the extracellular avenue of increased transepidermal water loss (TEWL) in both LI and loricrin keratoderma which provides definitive proof that the corneocyte provides the necessary scaffold for the supramolecular organization of the lipid-enriched, extracellular matrix.

A different mechanism is operative in EI (EHK), where abnormal keratins (either keratin 1 or 10) form dominant-negative keratin pairs that disrupt the cytoskeleton, thereby impeding lamellar body exocytosis [38]. Once again, the barrier abnormality in EHK is provoked via a defect in the extracellular matrix, i.e. a reduction in secreted lipids [38]. A similar pathogenic mechanism appears to occur in filaggrin-deficient mice that mimic certain mutations in ichthyosis vulgaris [39]. These mutations block the processing of profilaggrin into filaggrin, and unprocessed profilaggrin also appears to impede secretion of lamellar bodies. Thus, in inherited disorders of corneocyte proteins of diverse etiology, the protein abnormality ultimately provokes a defect in the *extracellular* lamellar membranes ('mortar') [7, 17, 37, 38]. This secondary defect in the extracellular matrix then allows accelerated, extracellular transcutaneous water movement, i.e. the permeability barrier abnormality, which 'drives' epidermal hyperplasia, results in a thickened (ichthyotic) SC.

1.6. Basis for Inflammation in the Ichthyoses

The SC serves as a biosensor, transmitting signals to the underlying nucleated, epidermal cell layers to initiate homeostatic repair responses, including both increased synthesis and secretion of lamellar body lipids, as well as stimulating epidermal

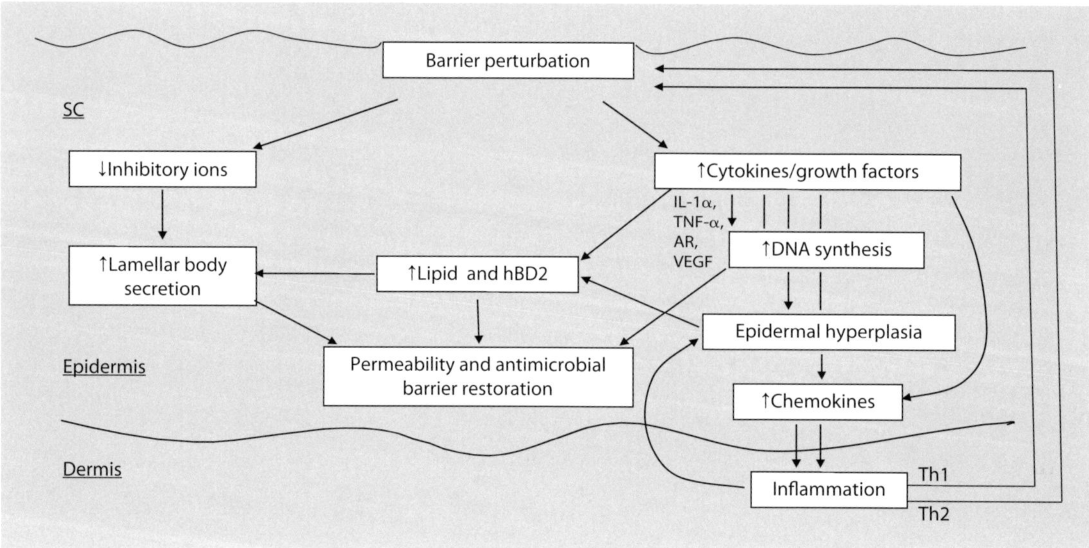

Fig. 10. Cytokine cascade due to altered barrier function leads to inflammation and further aggravates barrier dysfunction (modified from Elias et al. [42]). TNF-α = Tumor necrosis factor α; AR = amphiregulin; VEGF = vascular endothelial growth factor; hBD2 = type 2 β-defensin.

mitogenesis. Hence, the hyperplastic response aims to repair the barrier by providing both more corneocyte 'bricks', as well as additional keratinocytes that synthesize more lipids ('mortar') for the barrier. Yet, the homeostatic signaling mechanisms that attempt to restore barrier function also recruit downstream inflammatory mediators, and this results in the inflammation (erythema) that accompanies many of the ichthyoses [40–42]. When this cytokine cascade is sustained, both epidermal hyperplasia (with hyperkeratosis) and the inflammatory response are ongoing [41, 43], with further deterioration of barrier function by either Th1- and/or Th2-mediated mechanisms (fig. 10).

1.7. Basis for Abnormal Desquamation in the Ichthyoses

An additional major functional disturbance in the ichthyoses is abnormal desquamation. In normal SC, the gradual weakening of intercellular corneodesmosome attachments (fig. 11), through regulated proteolysis of these connectors, assisted by mechanical debridement, is thought to lead to invisible, mostly single-cell desquamation. This process is altered in all of the ichthyoses. The extent to which either dissolution of lamellar bilayers or the corneocyte lipid envelope contributes to normal intercorneocyte cohesion and conversely to the DOC and/or to normal desquamation remains unknown.

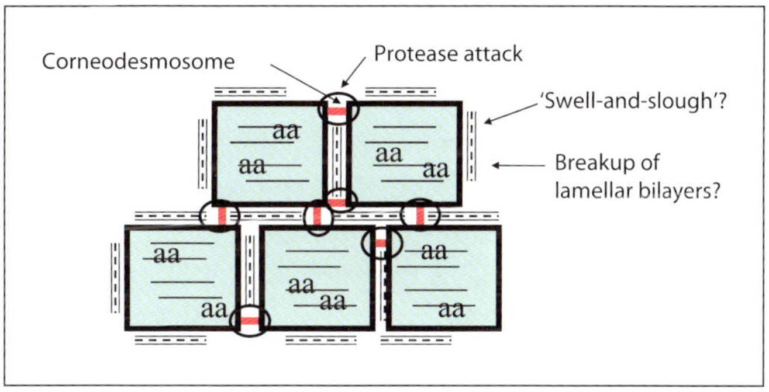

Fig. 11. Desquamation requires proteolysis of corneodesmosomes.

In any case, normal desquamation represents an orderly process, in which loss of corneocyte cohesion requires progressive proteolysis of corneodesmosomes [44–46] (fig. 11). To what extent changes in lamellar bilayer organization and/or 'swell-and-slough' associated with normal bathing [47] contribute to shedding of corneocytes remains unclear. The multiple protective functions of the epidermis require that SC not be shed prematurely. SC integrity/cohesion (SC integrity, i.e. resistance to shear forces, is experimentally defined as the rate of increase in TEWL with sequential tape stripping, and SC cohesion is defined as the quantity of protein removed per stripping), rely on corneodesmosomes, which form proteinaceous connections between adjacent corneocytes [48]. These structures are anchored into the cornified envelope by envoplakin and periplakin, while the intrinsic E-cadherins, desmoglein 1 and desmocollin 1, form homophilic bonds with their equivalents on opposing corneocytes [49]. The normal shedding of corneocytes is mediated by a cocktail of proteases, whose net activities vary according to depth-dependent changes in the pH of the SC [10, 50]. While normal SC is highly acidic at the skin surface (pH approx. 5), it becomes neutral near the stratum granulosum/SC interface [51, 52]. The external coat of corneodesmosomes, formed by corneodesmosin, is degraded initially by serine proteases (SP), which exhibit near-neutral pH optima [10, 53]. While SP activity is normally restricted to the lower SC, aspartate and cysteine proteases with acidic pH optima, such as the SC thiol protease and cathepsin D, are candidates to regulate desquamation in the outer SC [54]. However, in inflammatory dermatoses, including the ichthyoses, where pH remains abnormally elevated throughout the SC, it is likely that SP activity dominates at all levels [10].

Endogenous protease inhibitors are critically important to restrict protease activities such that corneodesmosome degradation does not occur prematurely. These inhibitors in the SC include the SP inhibitors, secretory leukocyte protease inhibitor, elafin, plasminogen activator inhibitor and lymphoepithelial Kazal-type inhibitor, type 1 (LEKTI-1), and the 2 cysteine protease inhibitors cystatin E/K and α [54]. Because all of these inhibitors (except LEKTI-1) possess TGM-1-binding domains, they incorporate to varying extents into the cornified envelope [54, 55], which is likely to make them less available to regulate SP-mediated proteolysis than LEKTI-1. The critical importance of LEKTI-1 is illustrated in NS [chapter 3, this vol., pp. 89–97], where the extent to which *LEKTI1* mutations result in loss of function correlates with: (1) the degree of SP activation, (2) the level of barrier dysfunction (resulting both from an unrestricted attack by SP on corneodesmosomes, with marked thinning of the SC, and from SP-mediated destruction of lipid-processing enzymes, with a failure to generate mature lamellar membranes) and (3) the severity of phenotype [56]. Moreover, once certain SP (i.e. KLK5) are activated, they can directly stimulate Th2 inflammation [57; chapter 3, this vol., pp. 89–97].

1.8. Systemic Consequences of Barrier Abnormalities in the Disorders of Cornification

In many patients with the severe generalized forms of ichthyosis (e.g. LI), heat intolerance occurs due to obstruction of sweat ducts. Certain ichthyoses are also accompanied by an increased susceptibility to cutaneous and systemic infections. A plausible scenario for these infectious complications is as follows. Certain SC lipids (e.g. free fatty acids) and antimicrobial peptides (the β-defensin hBD2 and the cathelicidin LL-37) are normally delivered by lamellar body secretion to the SC intercellular domains, and provide a first line of defense against microbial invasion. Failure of lamellar body secretion (e.g. in EI) or of lipid processing, required for the generation of free fatty acids (e.g. in NS), or proteolytic inactivation of antimicrobial peptides (e.g. in NS) may therefore account for the propensity for bacterial and fungal infections in EI, as well as bacterial and viral infections in NS [58–60].

Due to the energy losses that accompany evaporative water loss, infants and children with severe DOC can exhibit growth failure [61, 62], a phenomenon that is well recognized to occur in extensive thermal burns and in premature infants with immature skin barriers [63]. Short stature has been reported in some ichthyoses, such as NS [64], HI [65] and trichothiodystrophy [13, 65, 66], but growth failure can also occur in other DOC, including severe ARCI and EI phenotypes, implying that common pathogenic mechanism(s) are likely to be operative. While epidermal inflammation and hyperproliferation have previously been proposed to explain growth failure [67], negative nitrogen balance in adults does not occur until losses exceed 17 $g/m^2/day$ [68]. Therefore, nutrient losses from a hyperplastic epidermis are unlikely to account for growth failure in the DOC. Because transcutaneous evaporation is necessarily accompanied by loss of heat (0.58 kcal/ml) [69], excessive rates of TEWL can result in a significant caloric drain that if uncompensated would lead to impaired growth. Although all DOC subjects display impaired barrier function, TEWL rates vary widely, as would be expected in such a heterogeneous group of disorders. The number of kilocalories lost from daily total TEWL in one study of

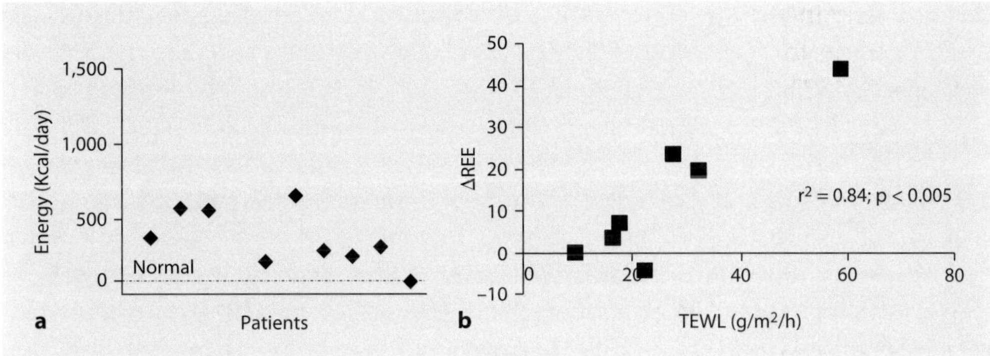

Fig. 12. **a** Energy losses due to increased TEWL. **b** Resting energy expenditure (REE) correlates with altered barrier function.

children with growth failure and a DOC ranged from 84 to 1,015 kcal/day (from 8 to 42 kcal/kg/day), with a mean of 433 ± 272 kcal/day, in contrast to expected rates of 41–132 kcal/day for children of comparable ages (fig. 12a). In those children with moderate to severe barrier abnormalities, barrier-related caloric losses were sufficient to account for their growth failure [62]. Moreover, barrier-related caloric losses could be compounded by additional caloric expenditures from excessive epidermal hyperplasia, chronic inflammation and/or anorexia accompanying systemic inflammation.

Children with the highest rates of TEWL also displayed the highest resting energy expenditures (fig. 12b), implying that the severity of the barrier defect correlates with increased metabolic demands. Some patients were in positive caloric balance at the time of study, but all had dropped below normal growth patterns early in life [61]. Hence, their positive caloric balance at the time of study likely reflected that they had eventually reached a steady state of growth. Nevertheless, they remained below normal body weight and/or height for their ages. Moreover, a significant number of these children were still in negative energy balance, suggesting how precariously even these older DOC patients maintain energy balance. Indeed, it is likely that infancy is a critical time for growth in these patients. Because growth rates are highest during the first year of life, infants with severe ichthyosis phenotypes are not able to compensate sufficiently for the combined caloric and fluid losses imposed by a defective barrier to support growth.

Assessment of the integrity of the lamellar bilayers and lamellar body secretory system was predictive of the barrier defect in this cohort. The severest barrier defects and ultrastructural abnormalities were observed in patients with HI and NS [62]. Finally, there can be other, unforeseen consequences of barrier failure in the DOC. Children with severe ichthyosis and growth failure are usually severely constipated and display hematocrits as well as serum Ca^{2+} and Mg^{2+} levels that are at or above the upper limits of normal [61], suggesting that fluid losses result in contraction of blood and extracellular fluid volumes (i.e. these patients are 'running dry').

1.9. Utility of Ultrastructure in the Differential Diagnosis of the Ichthyoses

Our previous studies on the cellular mechanisms that underlie the pathogenesis of the permeability barrier abnormality in the ichthyoses revealed the basis for the clinical phenotype in: (i) RXLI [70]; (ii) Chanarin-Dorfman syndrome (neutral lipid storage disease with ichthyosis) [71]; (iii) Gaucher disease [72]; (iv) TGM-1-negative LI [7]; (v) EI [38]; (vi) loricrin keratoderma (Vohwinkel syndrome) [37], and (vii) NS [56]. In this volume, we now demonstrate novel, ultrastructural features of ichthyosis vulgaris [Gruber, unpubl. data], Refsum disease, CHILD syndrome, Sjörgen-Larsson syndrome [73], IPS [74], neutral lipid storage disease with ichthyosis [75] below, and ichthyosis en confettis, which also help to explicate their disease phenotypes. During the course of these studies, certain disease-specific features emerged, which permit the provisional diagnosis of these disorders, within an appropriate clinical setting and pending confirmatory genotyping (table 4). These new images on genotyped patients include several startling new diagnostic features, such as loss of the corneocyte lipid envelope in Refsum disease and Chanarin-Dorfman syndrome, and evidence that 'uninvolved' skin sites in CHILD syndrome are actually 'involved'. We also have identified a unique complex of features in ichthyosis en confettis, which, although the genotype has not yet been published, should allow for diagnosis with a high degree of certainty (table 4). Finally, we also expand on prior ultrastructural studies on HI, showing here again how the failure to generate lamellar body contents leads to an absence of extracellular lamellar bilayers [35], but also reiterating that the corneocyte-bound lipid envelope, external to the cornified envelope, is normal. Thus, it is likely that secretion of *forme fruste* lamellar bodies in HI results in fusion of the organelles' limiting membrane with the plasma membrane, thereby forming the corneocyte lipid envelope [35].

Although the morphological features of most of these diseases are quite consistent, many characteristic alterations, such as the 'premature' secretion of lamellar bodies in NS, are not absolutely diagnostic (similar 'premature' secretion is also seen in psoriasis and some ARCI patients). Other ultrastructural abnormalities, such as lamellar/nonlamellar phase separation, although clear indicators of abnormal barrier function, occur in several of the ichthyoses, so in themselves they cannot be considered diagnostic. Nevertheless, in table 4, we highlight those features that are particularly helpful in the differential diagnosis of the ichthyoses. A final word of caution, we have no personal experience with the utility of cutaneous ultrastructure for the prenatal diagnosis of the ichthyoses. Because these structural features could differ during epidermal development in utero, it should not be assumed that the distinctive structural

Table 4. Ultrastructural diagnostic features of the ichthyoses

	KHG/ keratins	LB formation and contents	LB exocytosis	Lipid processing	Lamellar bilayers	Cornified envelopes	CD	CLE
Lipid metabolic								
ARCI (ichthyin)	normal/ normal	decreased	decreased	not assessed	not assessed	not assessed	normal	not assessed
ARCI *(ABCA12)*	decreased/ normal	*↓contents*	normal	n.a.	*largely absent*	normal	*persist*	*normal*
NLSDI	normal/ normal	*abnormal contents*	normal	normal	*L/non-L PS*	normal	normal	*abnormal*
SLS	normal/ normal	*cytolysis; abnormal contents*	*abnormal*	delayed	*L/non-L PS*	normal	normal	normal
Refsum	normal/ normal	*abnormal shape and contents*	*abnormal*	*delayed*	*L/non-L PS*	normal	*normal*	*absent*
CHH/ CHILD	normal/ normal	*abnormal contents*	*impaired*	*delayed*	*L/non-L PS*	normal	normal	normal
Gaucher	normal/ normal	normal	normal	*impaired*	*L/non-L PS*	normal	normal	normal
RXLI	normal/ normal	*normal*	normal	normal	*L/non-L PS*	normal	*persist*	*normal*
Lipid transporters								
HI	abnormal/ normal	*empty*	n.a.	n.a.	*absent*	normal	*persist*	
CEDNIK	?	empty	impaired	not assessed	not assessed	not assessed	not assessed	not assessed
IPS	normal/ normal	*abnormal contents*	normal	normal	*L/non-L PS*	normal	normal	normal
Structural proteins								
EI	*normal/ abnormal*	normal	*impaired*	*delayed*	*decreased/ fragmented*	persist	persist	normal
LI *(TGM1)*	normal/ normal	normal	normal	normal	*fragmented*	*absent/ attenuated*	normal	normal
LK	normal/ normal	normal	normal	normal	*fragmented*	*attenuated lower SC*	normal	normal
IV	*reduced/* normal	normal	*impaired*	*impaired*	*decreased, L/non-L PS*	normal	*persist*	*?abnormal*

Table 4. Continued

	KHG/ keratins	LB formation and contents	LB exocytosis	Lipid processing	Lamellar bilayers	Cornified envelopes	CD	CLE
Accelerated desquamation								
NS	normal/ abnormal	normal	*accelerated*	*impaired*	*reduced/ fragmented*	normal	*degraded*	*normal*
Other								
En confettis	*abnormal/ abnormal*	normal	*abnormal*	impaired	*decreased*	*absent*	*absent*	*normal*

Italicized features are particularly helpful in the differential diagnosis.
CD = Corneodesmosomes; CLE = corneocyte lipid envelope; KHG = keratohyalin granules; LB = lamellar body; CHH = Conradi-Hünermann-Happle syndrome; IV = ichthyosis vulgaris; LI = transglutaminase-1-deficient lamellar ichthyosis; LK = loricrin keratoderma (Vohwinkel); NLSDI = neutral lipid storage disease with ichthyosis (Chanarin-Dorfman syndrome); SLS = Sjögren-Larsson syndrome; L/non-L PS = lamellar/nonlamellar phase separation; n.a. = not applicable.

changes that we describe here for either children or adult DOC skin will necessarily be present in fetal epidermis.

1.10. References

1 Oji V, Tadini G, Akiyama M, et al: Revised nomenclature and classification of inherited ichthyoses: results of the first ichthyosis consensus conference in Sorèze 2009. J Am Acad Dermatol 2010, Epub, ahead of print.

2 Elias PM, Friend DS: The permeability barrier in mammalian epidermis. J Cell Biol 1975;65:180–191.

3 Elias PM, Goerke J, Friend DS: Mammalian epidermal barrier layer lipids: composition and influence on structure. J Invest Dermatol 1977;69:535–546.

4 Menon GK, Elias PM: Ultrastructural localization of calcium in psoriatic and normal human epidermis. Arch Dermatol 1991;127:57–63.

5 Raymond AA, Gonzalez de Peredo A, Stella A, et al: Lamellar bodies of human epidermis: proteomics characterization by high throughput mass spectrometry and possible involvement of CLIP-170 in their trafficking/secretion. Mol Cell Proteomics 2008;7:2151–2175.

6 Ishida-Yamamoto A, Kishibe M, Takahashi H, Iizuka H: Rab11 is associated with epidermal lamellar granules. J Invest Dermatol 2007;127:2166–2170.

7 Elias PM, Schmuth M, Uchida Y, et al: Basis for the permeability barrier abnormality in lamellar ichthyosis. Exp Dermatol 2002;11:248–256.

8 Potts RO, Francoeur ML: Lipid biophysics of water loss through the skin. Proc Natl Acad Sci USA 1990;87:3871–3873.

9 Uchida Y, Holleran WM, Elias PM: On the effects of topical synthetic pseudoceramides: comparison of possible keratinocyte toxicities provoked by the pseudoceramides, PC104 and BIO391, and natural ceramides. J Dermatol Sci 2008;51:37–43.

10 Elias PM: Stratum corneum defensive functions: an integrated view. J Invest Dermatol 2005;125:183–200.

11 Feingold KR: The regulation and role of epidermal lipid synthesis. Adv Lipid Res 1991;24:57–82.

12 Ghadially R, Brown BE, Sequeira-Martin SM, Feingold KR, Elias PM: The aged epidermal permeability barrier: structural, functional, and lipid biochemical abnormalities in humans and a senescent murine model. J Clin Invest 1995;95:2281–2290.

13 Traupe H: Ichthyosis: A Guide to Clinical Diagnosis, Genetic Counseling, and Therapy. New York, Springer, 1989, p 253.

14 Vahlquist A, Ganemo A, Pigg M, Virtanen M, Westermark P: The clinical spectrum of congenital ichthyosis in Sweden: a review of 127 cases. Acta Derm Venereol Suppl (Stockh) 2003;83:34–47.
15 Williams ML, Elias PM: From basketweave to barrier: unifying concepts for the pathogenesis of the disorders of cornification. Arch Dermatol 1993; 129:626–629.
16 Williams ML, Bruckner A, Nopper A: Generalized disorders of cornification (the ichthyoses); in Harper J, Orange A, Prose N (eds): Textbook of Pediatric Dermatology. Oxford, Blackwell Science, 2006, pp 1304–1358.
17 Schmuth M, Gruber R, Elias PM, Williams ML: Ichthyosis update: towards a function-driven model of pathogenesis of the disorders of cornification and the role of corneocyte proteins in these disorders. Adv Dermatol 2007;23:231–256.
18 Williams ML: Ichthyosis: mechanisms of disease. Pediatr Dermatol 1992;9:365–368.
19 Williams ML: Epidermal lipids and scaling diseases of the skin. Semin Dermatol 1992;11:169–175.
20 Di Giovanna JJ, Robinson-Bostom L: Ichthyosis: etiology, diagnosis, and management. Am J Clin Dermatol 2003;4:81–95.
21 Oji V, Traupe H: Ichthyoses: differential diagnosis and molecular genetics. Eur J Dermatol 2006;16:349–359.
22 Frost P, Weinstein GD, Van Scott EJ: The ichthyosiform dermatoses. II. Autoradiographic studies of epidermal proliferation. J Invest Dermatol 1966; 47:561–567.
23 Williams ML, Elias PM: The extracellular matrix of stratum corneum: role of lipids in normal and pathological function. Crit Rev Ther Drug Carrier Syst 1987;3:95–122.
24 Williams ML: Lipids in normal and pathological desquamation. Adv Lipid Res 1991;24:211–262.
25 Schmuth M, Jiang YJ, Dubrac S, Elias PM, Feingold KR: Thematic review series: skin lipids. Peroxisome proliferator-activated receptors and liver X receptors in epidermal biology. J Lipid Res 2008;49:499–509.
26 Oren A, Ganz T, Liu L, Meerloo T: In human epidermis, beta-defensin 2 is packaged in lamellar bodies. Exp Mol Pathol 2003;74:180–182.
27 Braff MH, Di Nardo A, Gallo RL: Keratinocytes store the antimicrobial peptide cathelicidin in lamellar bodies. J Invest Dermatol 2005;124:394–400.
28 Elias PM, Feingold KR: Stratum corneum barrier function: definitions and broad concepts; in Elias PM, Feingold KR (eds): Skin Barrier. New York, Taylor & Francis, 2006, pp 1–4.
29 Williams ML, Elias PM: Enlightened therapy of the disorders of cornification. Clin Dermatol 2003;21: 269–273.
30 Williams ML, Schmuth M, Crumrine D, et al: Pathogenesis of the ichthyoses: update and therapeutic implications. J Skin Barrier Res 2005;7:122–133.
31 Williams ML, Coleman RA, Placezk D, Grunfeld C: Neutral lipid storage disease: a possible functional defect in phospholipid-linked triacylglycerol metabolism. Biochim Biophys Acta 1991;1096:162–169.
32 Bouwstra JA, Ponec M: The skin barrier in healthy and diseased state. Biochim Biophys Acta 2006; 1758:2080–2095.
33 Williams ML, Elias PM: Genetically transmitted, generalized disorders of cornification: the ichthyoses. Dermatol Clin 1987;5:155–178.
34 Akiyama M: Pathomechanisms of harlequin ichthyosis and ABCA transporters in human diseases. Arch Dermatol 2006;142:914–918.
35 Elias PM, Fartasch M, Crumrine D, Behne M, Uchida Y, Holleran WM: Origin of the corneocyte lipid envelope (CLE): observations in harlequin ichthyosis and cultured human keratinocytes. J Invest Dermatol 2000;115:765–769.
36 Dale BA, Holbrook KA, Fleckman P, Kimball JR, Brumbaugh S, Sybert VP: Heterogeneity in harlequin ichthyosis, an inborn error of epidermal keratinization: variable morphology and structural protein expression and a defect in lamellar granules. J Invest Dermatol 1990;94:6–18.
37 Schmuth M, Fluhr JW, Crumrine DC, et al: Structural and functional consequences of loricrin mutations in human loricrin keratoderma (Vohwinkel syndrome with ichthyosis). J Invest Dermatol 2004; 122:909–922.
38 Schmuth M, Yosipovitch G, Williams ML, et al: Pathogenesis of the permeability barrier abnormality in epidermolytic hyperkeratosis. J Invest Dermatol 2001;117:837–847.
39 Scharschmidt TC, Man MQ, Hatano Y, et al: Filaggrin deficiency confers a paracellular barrier abnormality that reduces inflammatory thresholds to irritants and haptens. J Allergy Clin Immunol 2009;124:496–506, 506e1–6.
40 Elias PM: Stratum corneum architecture, metabolic activity and interactivity with subjacent cell layers. Exp Dermatol 1996;5:191–201.
41 Elias PM, Feingold KR: Does the tail wag the dog? Role of the barrier in the pathogenesis of inflammatory dermatoses and therapeutic implications. Arch Dermatol 2001;137:1079–1081.
42 Elias PM, Hatano Y, Williams ML: Basis for the barrier abnormality in atopic dermatitis: outside-inside-outside pathogenic mechanisms. J Allergy Clin Immunol 2008;121:1337–1343.

43 Elias PM, Wood LC, Feingold KR: Epidermal pathogenesis of inflammatory dermatoses. Am J Contact Dermatitis 1999;10:119–126.
44 Simon M, Montezin M, Guerrin M, Durieux JJ, Serre G: Characterization and purification of human corneodesmosin, an epidermal basic glycoprotein associated with corneocyte-specific modified desmosomes. J Biol Chem 1997;272:31770–3176.
45 Simon M, Jonca N, Guerrin M, et al: Refined characterization of corneodesmosin proteolysis during terminal differentiation of human epidermis and its relationship to desquamation. J Biol Chem 2001; 276:20292–20299.
46 Haftek M, Simon M, Kanitakis J, et al: Expression of corneodesmosin in the granular layer and stratum corneum of normal and diseased epidermis. Br J Dermatol 1997;137:864–873.
47 Williams ML: The ichthyoses – pathogenesis and prenatal diagnosis: a review of recent advances. Pediatr Dermatol 1983;1:1–24.
48 Haftek M, Simon M, Serre G: Corneodesmosomes: pivotal actors in the stratum corneum cohesion and desquamation; in Elias PM, Feingold KR (eds): Skin Barrier. New York, Taylor & Francis, 2006, pp 171–190.
49 Rawlings AV, Scott IR, Harding CR, Bowser PA: Stratum corneum moisturization at the molecular level. J Invest Dermatol 1994;103:731–741.
50 Brattsand M, Stefansson K, Lundh C, Haasum Y, Egelrud T: A proteolytic cascade of kallikreins in the stratum corneum. J Invest Dermatol 2005;124: 198–203.
51 Ohman H, Vahlquist A: In vivo studies concerning a pH gradient in human stratum corneum and upper epidermis. Acta Derm Venereol 1994;74:375–379.
52 Behne MJ, Meyer JW, Hanson KM, et al: NHE1 regulates the stratum corneum permeability barrier homeostasis: microenvironment acidification assessed with fluorescence lifetime imaging. J Biol Chem 2002;277:47399–47406.
53 Matsumoto M, Zhou Y, Matsuo S, et al: Targeted deletion of the murine corneodesmosin gene delineates its essential role in skin and hair physiology. Proc Natl Acad Sci USA 2008;105:6720–6724.
54 Zeeuwen PL: Epidermal differentiation: the role of proteases and their inhibitors. Eur J Cell Biol 2004; 83:761–773.
55 Steinert PM, Marekov LN: Initiation of assembly of the cell envelope barrier structure of stratified squamous epithelia. Mol Biol Cell 1999;10:4247–4261.
56 Hachem JP, Wagberg F, Schmuth M, et al: Serine protease activity and residual LEKTI expression determine phenotype in Netherton syndrome. J Invest Dermatol 2006;126:1609–1621.
57 Briot A, Deraison C, Lacroix M, et al: Kallikrein 5 induces atopic dermatitis-like lesions through PAR2-mediated thymic stromal lymphopoietin expression in Netherton syndrome. J Exp Med 2009; 206:1135–1147.
58 Sedlacek V, Krenar J: Symptomatology of Comel's linear circumflex ichthyosis (a case associated with genito-anal papillomatosis). Hautarzt 1971;22:390–397.
59 Folster-Holst R, Swensson O, Stockfleth E, Monig H, Mrowietz U, Christophers E: Comel-Netherton syndrome complicated by papillomatous skin lesions containing human papillomaviruses 51 and 52 and plane warts containing human papillomavirus 16. Br J Dermatol 1999;140:1139–1143.
60 Weber F, Fuchs PG, Pfister HJ, Hintner H, Fritsch P, Hoepfl R: Human papillomavirus infection in Netherton's syndrome. Br J Dermatol 2001;144:1044–1049.
61 Fowler AJ, Moskowitz DG, Wong A, Cohen SP, Williams ML, Heyman MB: Nutritional status and gastrointestinal structure and function in children with ichthyosis and growth failure. J Pediatr Gastroenterol Nutr 2004;38:164–169.
62 Moskowitz DG, Fowler AJ, Heyman MB, et al: Pathophysiologic basis for growth failure in children with ichthyosis: an evaluation of cutaneous ultrastructure, epidermal permeability barrier function, and energy expenditure. J Pediatr 2004;145:82–92.
63 Cartlidge P, Rutter N: Skin barrier function; in Polin R, Fox W (eds): Fetal and Neonatal Physiology. Philadelphia, Saunders, 1998, pp 771–788.
64 Greene SL, Muller SA: Netherton's syndrome: report of a case and review of the literature. J Am Acad Dermatol 1985;13:329–337.
65 Sybert VP: Genetic Skin Disorders. Oxford, Oxford University Press, 1997, pp 13–16, 205–208.
66 Williams M, Shwayder T: Ichthyosis and disorders of cornification; in Schachner LA, Hansen RC (eds): Pediatric Dermatology. New York, Churchill Livingstone, 1995, pp 413–454.
67 Judge MR, Morgan G, Harper JI: A clinical and immunological study of Netherton's syndrome. Br J Dermatol 1994;131:615–621.
68 Freedberg IM, Baden HP: The metabolic response to exfoliation. J Invest Dermatol 1962;38:277–284.
69 Perlstein P: Physical environment; in Fanaroff A, Martin R (eds): Neonatal-Perinatal Medicine. St Louis, Mosby Year Book, 1997, pp 481–501.
70 Elias PM, Crumrine D, Rassner U, Menon GK, Feingold KR, Williams ML: Pathogenesis of desquamation and permeability barrier abnormalities in RXLI; in Elias PM, Feingold KR (eds): Skin Barrier. New York, Taylor & Francis, 2006, pp 511–518.

71 Demerjian M, Crumrine DA, Milstone LM, Williams ML, Elias PM: Barrier dysfunction and pathogenesis of neutral lipid storage disease with ichthyosis (Chanarin-Dorfman syndrome). J Invest Dermatol 2006;126:2032–2038.
72 Holleran WM, Ginns EI, Menon GK, et al: Consequences of beta-glucocerebrosidase deficiency in epidermis: ultrastructure and permeability barrier alterations in Gaucher disease. J Clin Invest 1994; 93:1756–1764.
73 Rizzo WB, S'Aulis D, Jennings MA, Crumrine DA, Williams ML, Elias PM: Ichthyosis in Sjögren-Larsson syndrome reflects defective barrier function due to abnormal lamellar body structure and secretion. Arch Dermatol Res 2010, E-pub ahead of print.
74 Khnykin D, Crumrine D, Uchida Y, Jonansen F, Jahnsen F, Elias P: Epidermal barrier abnormalities and pathogenesis of ichthyosis prematurity syndrome. SID 2010 Annu Meet, Atlanta, 2010.
75 Uchida Y, Cho YH, Moradian S, et al: Neutral lipid storage leads to acylceramide deficiency, likely contributing to the pathogenesis of Dorman-Chanarin syndrome. SID 2010 Annu Meet, Atlanta 2010.

Inherited Clinical Disorders of Lipid Metabolism

An overview of the inherited lipid metabolic disorders with ichthyosis, which will be discussed in this chapter, is given in table 1.

2.1. Disorders of Fatty Acid Metabolism (Nonsyndromic)

2.1.1 Autosomal Recessive Congenital Ichthyoses

Background

The autosomal recessive congenital ichthyoses (ARCI), previously termed lamellar ichthyosis (LI), nonbullous congenital ichthyosiform erythroderma (CIE), or the LI/CIE spectrum, are a clinically and genetically heterogeneous group [1–5]. They all share in common an autosomal recessive mode of inheritance and disease presentation at birth, most often with a 'collodion membrane'. However, the neonatal phenotype can also range from generalized scaling to massive plate-like scales (the so-called harlequin fetus), while some have a 'cheesier', thickened stratum corneum (SC), likened to 'excessive vernix'. The phenotypes that subsequently evolve over the first few months of life can then also range from nearly normal skin (the so-called self-resolving collodion baby) to large plate-like scales (the LI phenotype) to marked erythema with fine, whitish scaling (the CIE phenotype). Some of the alterations in clinical phenotype that can occur over time are shown in figure 1.

The number of underlying genetic mutations is remarkable, with over 7 chromosomal loci implicated, of which 5 nonsyndromic ones have been identified to date [chapter 1, this vol., tables 2 and 3, pp. 6 and 8–9] (table 2, fig. 1) [6–14]. Moreover, a substantial fraction of patients do not have any of these mutations, suggesting that even greater genetic diversity exists. Before the genetic diversity within the ARCI spectrum became known, the LI phenotype, characterized by its large dark, plate-like scales, was distinguished clinically from nonbullous CIE or CIE, which typically displays fine scaling involving the flexures, as well as often prominent erythema [2]. Ultrastructural and biochemical differences between the LI and the CIE phenotypes provided initial clues about the heterogeneity within

Table 1. Inherited lipid metabolic disorders with ichthyosis

Metabolic category/ clinical disorder	Inheritance pattern	Multisystem	Affected protein and gene	Normal function
Fatty acid metabolism				
ARCI	autosomal recessive	no	12R-lipoxygenase *(ALOX12B)*	oxygenation of arachidonic acid to 12R-HPETE
ARCI	autosomal recessive	no	lipoxygenase 3 *(ALOXE3)*	hydroxyperoxide isomerization of 12R-HPETE to epoxy-alcohol metabolites
ARCI	autosomal recessive	no	cytochrome P450 *(CYP4F22, FLJ39501)*	?ω-hydroxylation of trioxilins
?ARCI	autosomal recessive	no	ichthyin (ichthyin)	unknown
Sjögren-Larsson syndrome	autosomal recessive	yes	fatty aldehyde dehydrogenase *(ALDH3A2)*	oxidation of fatty aldehydes to free fatty acids
Classic Refsum disease	autosomal recessive	yes	phytanoyl CoA hydroxylase *(PAHX, PHYH)*; peroxin 7 receptor *(PEX7)*	α-hydroxylation of plant-derived branched-chain FFA
Neutral lipid storage disease	autosomal recessive	yes	CGI-58 lipase activator *(ABHD5)*	generates DAG and FFA from TAG
Lipid transporter				
Harlequin ichthyosis	autosomal recessive	no	ATP-binding cassette *(ABCA12)*, loss of function	transports glucosylceramides into lamellar bodies
ARCI	autosomal recessive	no	ATP-binding cassette *(ABCA12)*, missense	see harlequin ichthyosis above
CEDNIK syndrome	autosomal recessive	yes	soluble N-ethyl-maleimide-sensitive factor attachment protein receptor *(SNAP29)*	facilitates exocytosis of lamellar body contents
Ichthyosis prematurity syndrome	autosomal recessive	no	fatty acid transport protein 4 *(FATP4)*	imports (?essential and/or long-chain) FFA

Table 1. Continued

Metabolic category/ clinical disorder	Inheritance pattern	Multisystem	Affected protein and gene	Normal function
Cholesterol metabolism				
Conradi-Hünermann-Happle syndrome	X-linked dominant	yes	Δ^8,Δ^7-sterol isomerase emopamil-binding protein *(EBP)*	distal cholesterol synthetic pathway
CHILD syndrome	X-linked dominant	yes	NAD(P)H steroid dehydrogenase-like protein *(NSDHL)*	distal cholesterol synthetic pathway
X-linked ichthyosis	X-linked recessive	(yes)	steroid sulfatase *(STS)*	desulfates sterol sulfates
Sphingolipid metabolism				
Gaucher disease type 1	autosomal recessive	yes	β-gluco-cerebrosidase *(GBA)*	deglucosylates glucosylceramides

ARCI = Autosomal recessive congenital ichthyosis; 12R-HPETE = 12R-hydroperoxyeicosatetraenoic acid; CoA = coenzyme A; FFA = free fatty acids; CGI-58 = comparative gene identification 58; DAG = diacylglyceride; TAG = triacylglyceride; CEDNIK = cerebral dysgenesis, neuropathy, ichthyosis and keratoderma; CHILD = congenital hemidysplasia with ichthyosiform erythroderma and limb defects.

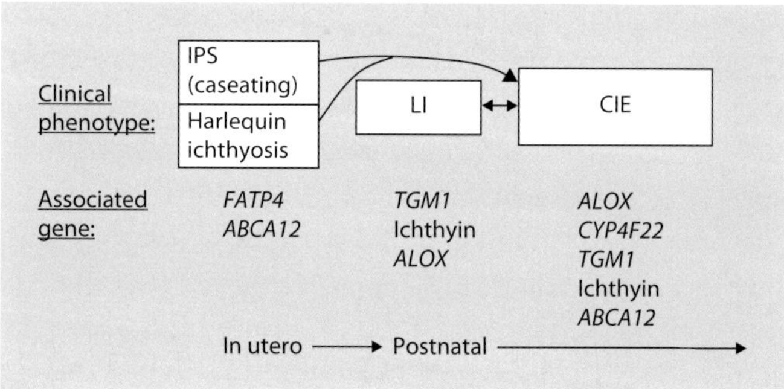

Fig. 1. Potential phenotypic shifts in the ARCI. IPS = Ichthyosis prematurity syndrome.

this group of ichthyoses [2, 4, 15], but intermediate phenotypes were also recognized [16, 17].

Several recently discovered mutations that cause ARCI encode enzymes that are directly involved in the synthesis, transport or assembly of lipid components of the SC (table 2; fig. 2, 3). Moreover, the LI phenotype is often predictive of a transglutaminase 1 *(TGM1)* mutation that assembles the chymotryptic enzyme; hence it is not

Table 2. Genotype-phenotype correlation within the ARCI spectrum

Clinical subtypes	Genes	OMIM No.
Harlequin ichthyosis	*ABCA12*	242500
Lamellar ichthyosis	*TGM1*	242300
	ABCA12	601277
	Ichthyin	609383
	12p11–13	not yet given
Bathing suit ichthyosis	*TGM1*	242300
Self-resolving collodion baby	*TGM1*	242300
	ALOXE3/ALOX12	242100
Congenital ichthyosiform erythroderma	*ALOXE3/ALOX12*	242100
	TGM1	242300
	Ichthyin	609383
	CYP4F22	604777
	ABCA12	601277
Congenital ichthyosis with fine/focal scaling	Ichthyin	609383
	CYP4F22	604777

a primary lipid abnormality. However, missense ATP-binding cassette A12 *(ABCA12)* mutations can also produce a severe LI phenotype [20, 21]. Conversely, *TGM1* mutations can underlie CIE phenotypes, as well as the bathing suit ichthyosis and the self-resolving collodion baby [22, 23]. Because of this overlap of phenotypes and genotypic complexities, the acronym ARCI was recently introduced as an umbrella term for these disorders [chapter 1, this vol., pp. 1–29]. Although several other syndromic, recessive ichthyoses can present at birth and thereafter with often similar phenotypes, e.g. Sjögren-Larsson syndrome (SLS), Gaucher disease (GD) or neutral lipid storage disease with ichthyosis (NLSDI), the term ARCI is currently reserved for nonsyndromic traits.

Clinical Features

Hopes for distinctive genotype-phenotype correlations – as new causative genes have been identified within the LI/CIE spectrum – have been largely disappointing. ARCI is almost always congenital, with newborns usually, but not always, covered by a thickened, taut SC, the so-called collodion membrane that transforms into generalized scaling of varying severity and variable degrees of erythroderma within the first few weeks of life [24]. In most instances, involvement is generalized, including the face, flexures and palms/soles. As stated earlier, a spectrum of phenotypes is recognized, ranging from those with thick plate-like scales (LI phenotype) at one pole to finer scaling, often with marked erythroderma (CIE) at the other, but there are

Table 3. Ichthyoses that have (or likely have) lamellar/nonlamellar phase separation

Disease	Enzymatic defect	Abnormal barrier function	Lamellar/ nonlamellar phase separation	Likely phase-separated lipid
Neutral lipid storage disease	neutral lipid hydrolase (CGI-58)	↑TEWL demonstrated[1]	demonstrated[1]	triglycerides (cited[1])
Recessive X-linked ichthyosis	steroid sulfatase	↑TEWL demonstrated[2]	demonstrated[2]	cholesterol sulfate
Refsum disease	phytanoyl-CoA hydroxylase (PHYH); peroxin 7 receptor	not known	shown here	phytanic acid in all glycerolipids[3]
Sjögren-Larsson syndrome	fatty aldehyde dehydrogenase	shown here by lanthanum perfusion	demonstrated[4,5]	assessed
Gaucher disease, type 2	β-gluco-cerebrosidase	↑TEWL demonstrated (lanthanum)[6]	demonstrated[6]	glucosyl-ceramides[6]
CHILD syndrome	NAD(P)H 3β-hydroxysteroid dehydrogenase (NSDHL)	shown here by lanthanum perfusion	shown here	not assessed
Conradi-Hünermann-Happle syndrome	Δ^8,Δ^7-sterol isomerase emopamil-binding protein (EBP)	not assessed	demonstrated[7]	not assessed
Ichthyosis prematurity syndrome	fatty acid transporter 4 (FATP4)	shown by lanthanum perfusion[8]	demonstrated[8]	not assessed

TEWL = Transepidermal water loss; CHILD = congenital hemidysplasia with ichthyosiform erythroderma and limb defects; CoA = coenzyme A.
[1] Demerjian et al. [66], 2006.
[2] Elias et al. [94], 2004.
[3] Van den Brink and Wanders [95], 2006.
[4] Shibaki et al. [96], 2004.
[5] Rizzo [97], 2007.
[6] Holleran et al. [98], 2006.
[7] Emami et al. [99], 1994.
[8] Khnykin et al. [100], 2010.

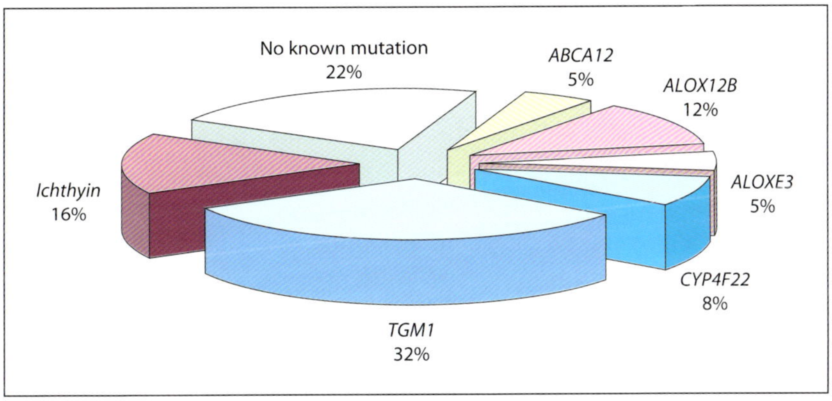

Fig. 2. Distribution of mutations in a cohort of 520 ARCI patients (from Fischer [18], with permission).

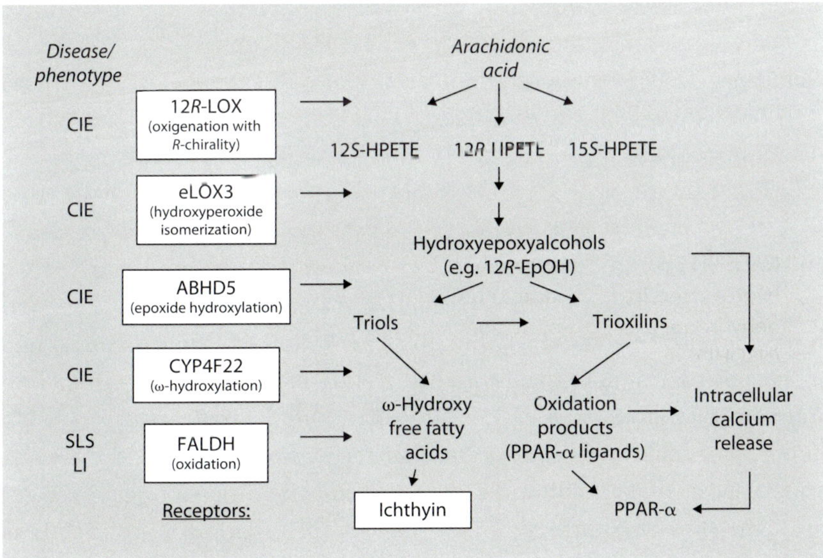

Fig. 3. Putative pathways whereby inherited abnormalities of lipid metabolism could lead to ichthyosis (modified from Elias et al. [19]). SLS = Sjögren-Larsson syndrome; HPETE = hydroperoxyeicosatetraenoic acid; EpOH = hydroxyepoxyalcohol; PPAR = peroxisome proliferator-activated receptor.

many intermediate phenotypes, and the phenotype can shift both at birth and during postnatal development (fig. 1). Facial tautness can result in eclabium and ectropion, with incomplete closure of the eyelids (lagophthalmus), leading to conjunctivitis and keratitis, which is often severest in the neonatal period. However, in severer phenotypes, it can be present throughout life. Palmar-plantar keratoderma is present with severity that usually parallels the skin disorder. In some cases, nail abnormalities and scalp involvement can lead to alopecia, often exacerbated by dermatophyte infections. Finally, hypohidrosis, complicated by heat intolerance, is a common complication.

Several clinical variants are recognized. Some patients resolve almost completely after birth. These so-called self-resolving or self-improving collodion babies may have one of several genes implicated, including *ALOXE3*, *ALOX12B* and *TGM1* [21–23]. Ichthyosis prematurity syndrome (IPS) also changes postnatally from an in utero, excessive vernix-like phenotype into a much milder CIE-like phenotype. This disorder is caused by loss-of-function mutations in the fatty acid transporter type 4 (FATP4) [25]. Harlequin ichthyosis (HI) is another recognized subset of ARCI, typically presenting at birth with massive, restrictive plate-like scales, accompanied by marked ectropion, eclabium and digital constrictions. HI infants that survive the neonatal period go on to develop a severe, erythrodermic CIE-like phenotype. HI is due to loss-of-function mutations in *ABCA12*, while missense mutations instead cause a less severe LI phenotype, which may be more common than is currently appreciated [26]. Finally, the so-called bathing suit ichthyosis where lamellar scaling is confined to the trunk, has been seen to date only with certain *TGM1* mutations.

The term 'collodion' describes a parchment/cellophane/plastic-wrap-like membrane covering the whole body surface [27, 28]. The 'collodion baby' phenotype is not specific to ARCI but can be seen in a variety of syndromic disorders of cornification (DOC), including SLS, recessive X-linked ichthyosis (RXLI), neonatal GD and even in non-DOC traits, such as ectodermal dysplasia. Conversely, a lack of a history of a congenital collodion membrane does not preclude the diagnosis of ARCI; affected neonates, particularly with ichthyin mutations, can also present with generalized erythema and scaling. Moreover, clear documentation of neonatal presentation is often lacking in individual cases. Thus, there is no reliable information about the relative frequency of a collodion membrane versus other neonatal phenotypes in ARCI. Furthermore, at least 2 autosomal dominant traits, loricrin keratoderma and ichthyosis en confettis, can present initially with cutaneous features of CIE. However, the systemic manifestations of several of the syndromic DOC can be either subtle or of delayed onset (e.g. GD type 2, NLSDI, Netherton syndrome, trichothiodystrophy, ichthyosis follicularis/alopecia/photophobia syndrome and sometimes RXLI). Hence, until the causative gene in an individual has been identified, the diagnosis of ARCI must be considered as only provisional.

Biochemical Genetics

Although the variability of the ARCI phenotype can be explained in part by genetic heterogeneity, it is also apparent that some reported ultrastructural findings reflect nonspecific sequelae of disturbed cornification. Thus, newly discovered gene mutations do not always correlate well or explain the observed clinical and morphological phenotypes; e.g. the LI phenotype is frequently, but not exclusively, caused by TGM-1 deficiency, i.e. the LI phenotype can result from mutations other than *TGM1* (fig. 3), and conversely, TGM-1 deficiency can produce other phenotypes (table 2) [11,

29–31]. Nevertheless, in an intense, ongoing effort, including structural correlations, detailed genotype-phenotype relationships are currently being developed [5, 18]. For example, the consequences of mutations in ichthyin (a putative transmembrane receptor, encoded on chromosome 5q33) on epidermal ultrastructure have been studied with standard electron microscopy [32] (see below).

Since a substantial fraction (>20%) of patients with ARCI phenotypes lack mutations of any known causative genes [18], it seems likely that additional causative genes may be identified in the future. For example, deficiency of the thiol protease inhibitor cystatin M/E could account for or contribute to the pathogenesis of some of these patients [33]. Although normal cystatin M/E expression is observed in the stratum granulosum (SG) in most cases of LI, including those showing TGM-1 deficiency, as well as in both ichthyosis vulgaris and HI, 3 patients with an LI phenotype displayed reduced immunostaining for cystatin M/E [34]. One of these patients presented with enhanced expression of cystatin M/E associated with a single mutation in exon 1 (AA110TT), which results in a shift from glutamic acid to valine (E37V) adjacent to the active site of this proteinase inhibitor [34]. This severely affected patient was also heterozygous for a profilaggrin mutation, a major predisposing factor of ichthyosis vulgaris and atopic dermatitis. While single-allele profilaggrin mutations typically cause mild disease, this patient had a severe ichthyosiform phenotype, suggesting that loss-of-function mutations in cystatin M/E combined with single-allele reduced function in filaggrin could account for this patient's severe phenotype. This highly instructional case further underscores the hazard of assigning a mode of inheritance (implicit in the term ARCI) before the patient has been genotyped.

Pathogenic Considerations

Lesueur et al. [31] have proposed that a single pathogenic pathway may underlie a number of the ARCI, a well as several of the syndromic DOC. The endogenous ligands for the putative ichthyin receptor are ω-hydroxyepoxyalcohols [30], presumably generated within normal epidermis [35] and reportedly esterified at high rates into phospholipids [36]. Epidermal hydroxyepoxyalcohols are themselves metabolic products of 12R-lipoxygenase (LOX) and hydroperoxide isomerase (epoxyalcohol synthase) eLOX3 [37, 38] (fig. 3). Mutations in *ALOX12B* and *ALOXE3* on chromosome 17p13, which result in a complete loss of enzymatic activity due to abnormal protein folding, are relatively common (>10%) among patients with ARCI [9, 12, 31, 39] (fig. 2). These enzymes catabolize leukotriene derivatives of arachidonic acid to 12R-hepoxilin A3 and 12R-hydroperoxyeicosatetraenoic acid [38, 39] (fig. 3). That this pathway has important relevance for the permeability barrier is shown by *12R-Alox* knockout (ko) mice, which display increased transepidermal water loss and early postnatal death [40, 41].

Several intermediate metabolic steps of this pathway could also produce an ARCI phenotype and permeability barrier abnormalities [31, 42] (fig. 1). First, some ARCI pedigrees linked to *ALOX12B/ALOXE3* lack mutations in these genes, suggesting that there could be an additional gene(s) in this region that encode(s) a protein within the same pathway [31]. Second, in other ARCI kindreds, mutations in cytochrome P450, family 4, subfamily F, polypeptide 22 *(CYP4F22)* on chromosome 19p12, encode a putative fatty acid ω-hydroxylase. It has been proposed that this enzyme could be responsible for an event late in the epoxyalcohol oxidation-hydroxylation cascade (fig. 3) [43]. Third, fatty aldehyde dehydrogenase (FALDH), which is deficient in SLS, may also oxidize trioxilin products within the above pathway.

However, it must be emphasized that none of these purported links to the trioxilin pathway has been experimentally confirmed [44]. Moreover, prominent CNS abnormalities occur in SLS, which are lacking in other ARCI phenotypes, indicating that the pathophysiological consequences of blockade at this step are much broader in scope. Furthermore, differences in the cutaneous phenotype of SLS (a 'lichenified' rather than 'scaly' pattern, accompanied by prominent pruritus) suggest that additional substrates could be affected. It has been further proposed that comparative gene identification 58 (*CGI58)*/α/β-hydrolase domain-containing 5 (*ABHD5),* which is mutated in patients with the multisystem disorder NLSDI, could also function as an epoxide hydroxylase in the same pathway [43], but the activities of this lipase are likely not restricted to these epoxide metabolites, because labeling studies suggest broader alterations in glycerolipid metabolism [45, 46]. Thus, while a unitary hypothesis is always attractive [31], it should be recalled that mutations in disparate genes, such as *TGM1* (see above), can cause identical phenotypes. Thus, it is likely that any derangement of epidermal lipid metabolism can provoke an ichthyosiform phenotype through effects on the permeability barrier and downstream consequences of a defective barrier, and therefore it may not be necessary to invoke a single metabolic pathway.

The pathogenesis of epoxide pathway defects could also be related to that of essential fatty acid deficiency, where deficiency of the substrate for ω-esterification, i.e. linoleic acid, to acylceramide is known to provoke a barrier abnormality [47–50]. Alternatively, some of the accumulating hydroxyepoxyalcohol substrates are potent and selective activators of the peroxisome proliferator-activated receptor, PPAR-α [51], a ligand-activated nuclear hormone receptor with prodifferentiating and anti-inflammatory activities in the epidermis [52–56] (fig. 3). In addition, CYP4F22 activity likely also generates potent endogenous PPAR-α activators, since it is a homologue of the leukotriene B_2/ω-hydroxylase, and ω-hydroxylation of other eicosanoids enhances PPAR-α-activating properties [43, 57]. Yet, the biological significance of this potential role remains unclear, since loss of PPAR-α only results in transient developmental defects in fetal mouse epidermis [55], presumably due to the redundant action of other epidermal nuclear hormone receptors. Finally, one or more of these metabolites could mobilize intracellular calcium, thereby altering permeability barrier homeostasis by downregulating lamellar body secretion [52, 58]. The last possibility is consistent with the lamellar body secretory defect that has been described in preliminary studies of this group of ichthyoses (e.g. ichthyin mutations, see below).

Finally, *ABC12* mutations that leave residual enzymatic function yield a milder LI phenotype, likely due to a lesser lamellar body secretory abnormality than occurs in HI itself [26].

Distinctive Ultrastructural Features

A functional barrier abnormality is present in all ARCI subtypes studied to date [59, 60], but the basis of the barrier abnormality is not known. Most ARCI phenotypes (with normal TGM-1) display prominent abnormalities in lamellar body, as well as in SC extracellular lamellar membrane structure. While the density of lamellar bodies is increased, many organelles are smaller than normal and display fragmented lamellar contents, often imparting to them a vacuolated appearance [4]. Thus, disorganized lamellar arrays and nonlamellar/lamellar phase separation appear to account for the barrier abnormality [4]. Recent studies in *Aloxe3* and *Alox12b* ko mice may shed light on these mechanisms. *Alox12b* ko mouse epidermis, transplanted on to SCID mice, displays defective profilaggrin processing [61] as well as altered ceramide metabolism [40]. The reported decrease in bound ω-OH ceramides could reflect either a loss of, or an abnormality in, the cornified lipid envelope, but this possibility has not yet been examined.

Several variable ultrastructural features have been observed in subsets of ARCI patients, including: (1) absence of electron-lucent lamellae; (2) abnormal spacing and interruptions of lamellar structures, and (3) intracellular lipid droplets and vesicular complexes, both within corneocytes and SG cells [4, 15, 59, 62, 63]. A classification of the ultrastructural findings in ARCI is still commonly utilized in Europe: type 1, characterized by abundant lipid droplets within corneocytes; type 2 showing polygonal clefts within the SC; type 3 showing vesicular and membranous structures in the SG, and type 4 characterized by lentiform swollen areas within corneocytes and perinuclear accumulation of curved membranes in the SG [3, 15]. While this classification has been somewhat useful diagnostically, it preceded the utilization of ruthenium tetroxide (RuO_4) postfixation [chapter 1, this vol., pp. 1–29].

On electron microscopy, the SG of patients with ichthyin mutations contains many empty or partially filled vacuolar and vesicular structures, which are thought to represent defective lamellar bodies [32]. Conversely, 85% of patients with this morphological pattern have mutations in ichthyin [32]. Patients with *ABCA12* missense mutations display lamellar bodies that lack an orderly membranous content intermingled with normal-appearing lamellar bodies in the upper spinous and granular cell layers [64]. Ultrastructural examination of mice with 12R-lox deficiency reveals vesicular structures in upper SG cells [64] that are comparable to reported structural abnormalities in human ARCI subjects with ichthyin mutations [32]. These mice also display an increase in protein-bound, ester-linked lipid species [40]. Finally, corneocytes isolated from 12R-lox-deficient animals are more fragile and show abnormal filaggrin processing [40], again features that have not yet been assessed in affected human skin. While the ultrastructure of other genetically defined ARCI subsets is currently unknown, abnormalities in ARCI due to *TGM1* deficiency are described in chapter 4 [this vol., pp. 98–127].

2.2. Multisystem Diseases of Fatty Acid Metabolism

2.2.1 Neutral Lipid Storage Disease with Ichthyosis (Chanarin-Dorfman Syndrome)

Clinical Diagnosis

Neonates with NLSDI, or Chanarin-Dorfman syndrome (OMIM No. 275630), typically present with an erythroderma with small whitish scales or less frequently as a collodion baby. Although the ichthyosiform phenotype in NLSDI is nondiagnostic, it most closely resembles ARCI [65, 66]. Yet, some NLSDI patients also display intense pruritus, with or without atopic features [66, 67], or an erythrokeratoderma-variabilis-like [68] or a severe 'oily' (seborrheic) phenotype [69], features that are not typically present in the ARCI. Triacylglycerol accumulation in cytosolic droplets in multiple tissues allows rapid clinical diagnosis of NLSDI by oil red O staining of frozen tissue sections from either skin or muscle or in peripheral blood smears. In skin biopsies, these droplets localize both to the epidermal basal layer and to appendageal epithelia [65] as well as within fibroblasts and other dermal cells. Lipid vacuoles can be readily demonstrated in polymorphonuclear leukocytes, eosinophils and monocytes on blood smears [65, 67]. Systemic symptoms and signs are usually present, including hepatosplenomegaly, steatorrhea, cataracts, neurosensory deafness, subtle muscle weakness, short stature and mild developmental delay, but these can be subtle. Hence, examination of a peripheral blood smear for lipid vacuoles is recommended for all patients with ARCI phenotypes [65, 67].

Biochemical Genetics

NLSDI is a rare disorder, largely occurring in consanguineous families of Mediterranean or Middle Eastern origin that is usually due to recessive homozygous or rarely compound heterozygous mutations in the gene encoding *ABHD5* (also known as *CGI58*). *CGI58/ABHD5* is located on chromosome 3p21, has 7 exons and its translation product is expressed in many tissues, including the skin. Loss of *CGI58* function leads to accumulation of cytosolic triacylglycerides (TAG), and the extent of TAG accumulation has recently been shown to correlate with severity of the dermatosis [70]. *CGI58* encodes for a 349-amino-acid protein that coactivates adipose triglyceride lipase, initiating hydrolysis of TAG into diacylglycerides, monoglycerides and free fatty acids (FFA). In contrast, desnutrin (*PNPLA2* or *TTS22* [68, 71–73]) encodes a protein that functions as the activator of a newly identified adipose triglyceride lipase, a lipase that is largely restricted to adipose tissue [74]. Thus, loss of adipose triglyceride lipase function is not associated with ichthyosis, but rather a lipid storage myopathy [46, 75, 76]. Therefore, *ABHD5* could activate a different lipase that is present in multiple tissues, including epidermis.

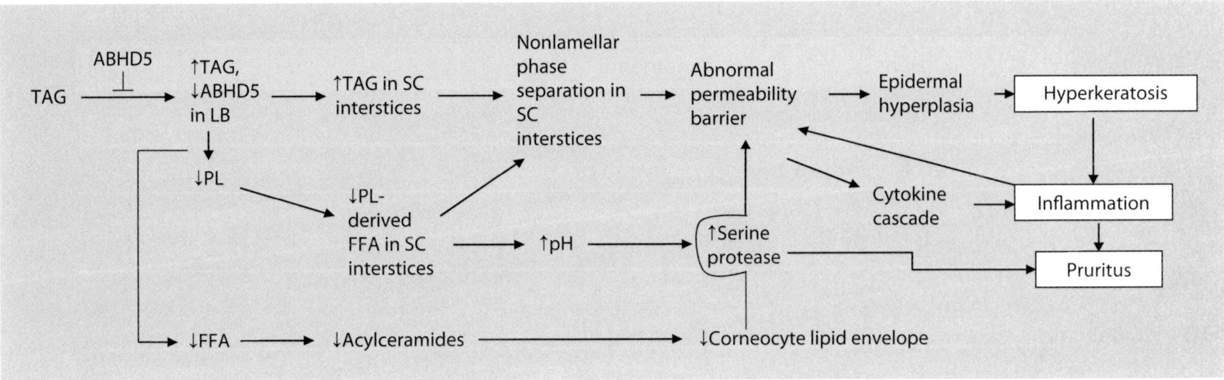

Fig. 4. Proposed pathogenic mechanisms in NLSDI. LB = Lamellar bodies; PL = phospholipids.

Cellular Pathogenesis

While the pathway that leads to cytosolic TAG accumulation in NLSDI has not been fully characterized, labeling studies suggest that the affected pool of TAG normally provides a rapidly turning-over reservoir of FFA utilized first for phospholipid synthesis [45, 77, 78], but recent studies in NLSDI and in *Cgi58* ko mice suggest that TAG accumulation also reduces the bioavailability of fatty acids for acylceramide production, consistent with our very recent observations that the corneocyte lipid envelope is absent in NLSDI [76] (see below).

If reduced bioavailability of diacylglycerol results in a failure of phospholipid synthesis and loading into lamellar bodies, this could provide an additional mechanism contributing to the barrier abnormality (fig. 4). Deficiency of secreted phospholipids would result in a downstream deficiency of FFA in that all secreted phospholipids are hydrolyzed to FFA that are one of the three key lipid constituents of the extracellular lamellar bilayers in normal SC [79]. Moreover, phospholipid-derived FFA also acidify normal SC [80]; hence, the pH of SC could also be elevated in NLSDI. An elevated pH in turn could activate serine proteases, which would contribute both to the barrier abnormality and provoke the intense pruritus that occurs in many NLSDI patients (fig. 4) [81]. Finally, as proposed by Lefevre et al. [71], *CGI58/ABHD5* could also catalyze epoxide hydroxylation (fig. 3) and contribute to disease phenotype in NLSDI in a manner similar to other ARCI (see above).

Neutral lipid-positive storage vacuoles likely do not account for the barrier abnormality in NLSDI, because these large, cytosolic inclusions become entombed within corneocytes, where they are unavailable to influence either permeability barrier homeostasis or desquamation. Moreover, comparable cytosolic lipid droplets occur as a nonspecific response to toxic insults and are seen in many hyperplastic dermatoses [82–86]. Likely more pertinent to disease phenotype in NLSDI are the lipid micro-inclusions that occur within epidermal lamellar bodies [65] (see below). In normal

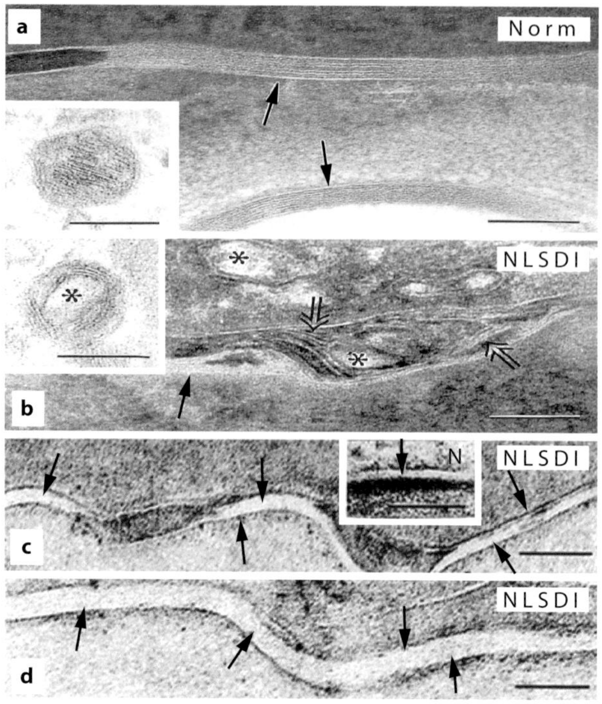

Fig. 5. Ultrastructure of SC in NLSDI. Key ultrastructural features: (1) microvesicles within lamellar bodies (**b**, inset, asterisk); (2) lamellar/nonlamellar phase separation (**b**, open arrows; asterisks = nonlamellar material); (3) absent corneocyte lipid envelope (**c**, **d**, arrows). Magnification bars = 0.1 μm.

epidermis, lamellar bodies are replete with lamellar membranes that show little or no evidence of nonlamellar discontinuities (fig. 5) [chapter 1, this vol., fig. 5, p. 14]. Following secretion, these lamellar contents then transform into 'mature' lamellar membrane structures that again fill the SC interstices [87], forming a uniform lamellar phase that completely fills the SC interstices (fig. 5a). In NLSDI, lamellar-body-containing vesicular inclusions are secreted, along with normal-appearing lamellar membranes, at the SG/SC interface [65]. Pertinently, in normal epidermis, lamellar bodies encapsulate the *CGI58/ABHD5* co-activator [72, 88]. In NLSDI, however, the co-activator protein is reduced or absent, and its lipid substrate accumulates, likely leading to disease pathogenesis (fig. 4).

Permeability barrier function is markedly abnormal in NLSDI, with basal transepidermal water loss levels up to 3-fold higher than in age-matched, normal controls [66], with severity comparable to other ichthyoses with a similar phenotype, such as TGM-1-deficient ARCI [59, 89]. Together, these studies suggest that persistence of secreted, 'unprocessed' TAG, coupled with decreased FFA, is one contributor to the functional abnormalities in NLSDI (fig. 4). In addition, our very recent studies suggest that the corneocyte lipid envelope is absent in NLSDI, a finding that correlates with decreased acylceramide synthesis [76, 90] (fig. 5c, d).

To assess definitively whether an inhomogeneous extracellular matrix forms an inherently less effective permeability barrier than normal interstices that are uniformly replete with lamellar membranes, we perfused the SC of NLSDI with a water-soluble, electron-dense tracer, lanthanum nitrate. While the interstices of normal human SC completely exclude water-soluble molecules, in NLSDI, lanthanum permeated through the nonlamellar domains in the extracellular spaces at all levels of the SC [66]. In summary, these studies show that lamellar/nonlamellar phase separation and acylceramide deficiency underlie the permeability barrier abnormality in NLSDI.

Diagnostic Ultrastructure and the Concept of Phase Separation
In NLSDI, lamellar bodies instead display vesicular microinclusions that transform into phase-separated (nonlamellar) lipid (fig. 5b, inset). With RuO_4 postfixation, the nonlamellar phase appears filled with an amorphous, electron-lucent material, which lies interspersed within short arrays of lamellar membranes [66] (fig. 5b). Classically, phase separation occurs in phospholipid-based membrane bilayers, when the amount of nonpolar lipid exceeds the capacity for the excess lipid to incorporate into polar lipid-based membranes [91], but in SC membranes, phase separation can also occur when certain polar lipids exceed the carrying capacity of membranes, as with cholesterol sulfate in RXLI and with excess glucosylceramide in type 2 GD [92, 93] (table 3; see also below). The frequent occurrence of nonlamellar phase separation in those ichthyoses associated with lipid metabolic disorders suggests that the ceramide-based membrane bilayers of normal SC also display a limited capacity to incorporate both excess nonpolar lipid species, such as triacylglycerols in NLSDI, and the excess polar species in RXLI and GD. Together, the combination of lamellar/nonlamellar phase separation, microvesicles within lamellar bodies and the absence of the corneocyte lipid envelope is diagnostic of NLSDI.

2.2.2 Sjögren-Larsson Syndrome

Clinical Features
Patients with SLS (OMIM No. 270200) display a characteristic triad of mild-to-profound mental retardation, spastic di- or tetraplegia and congenital ichthyosis [97, 101]. Neonates may present with a collodion membrane and erythema, which rapidly disappear, leaving the characteristic dermatosis; or they may present with exaggerated neonatal desquamation [102]. Once established, the epidermal phenotype is quite characteristic, exhibiting extreme pruritus and ridged or 'lichenified' skin, with fine, brown desquamation. Flexures are typically disproportionately involved, and periumbilical striations are also common [103]. The extreme pruritus has been attributed to accumulation of the proinflammatory leukotriene metabolite leukotriene B_4 [97, 104], but the possibility of a barrier defect leading to serine-protease-stimulated pruritus, with a Th2 phenotype, should also be considered. While the histopathology of SLS demonstrates nonspecific features, such as papillated epidermal hyperplasia and

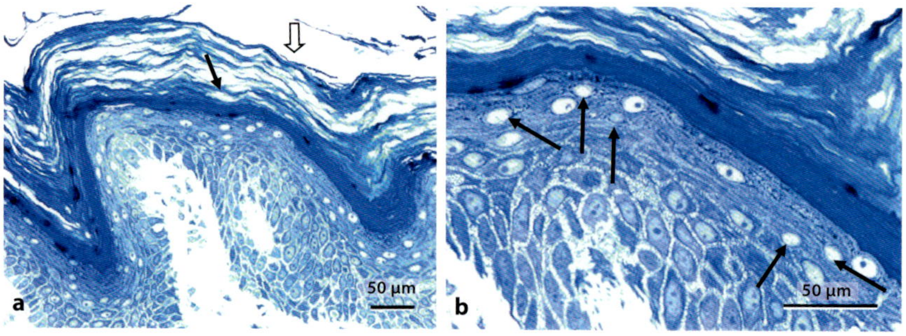

Fig. 6. Histopathology of SLS. **a** At low magnification, epidermal hyperplasia, spongiosis and prominent hyperkeratosis are evident. Note compactness of lower SC (solid arrow) and loosely organized mid to upper SC (open arrow). **b** At higher magnification, the granular layer (arrows) is normal in size, but some individual cells appear vacuolated. Epon embedded, 1-µm section, toluidine blue staining. Magnification bars = 50 µm.

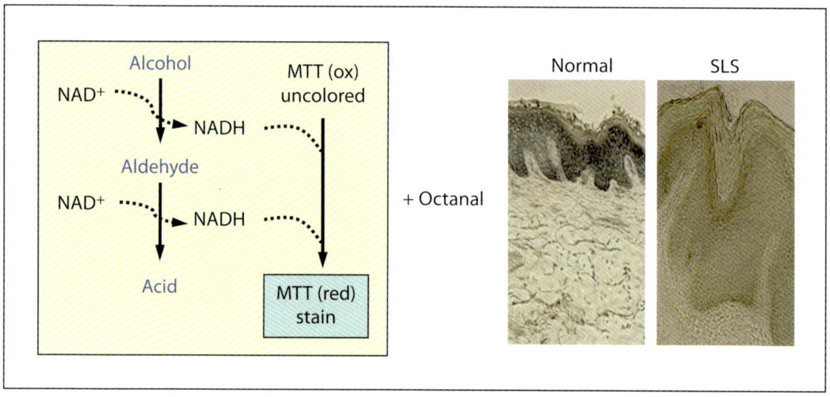

Fig. 7. Histochemical staining for FALDH activity (courtesy of William Rizzo, MD).

hyperkeratosis, closer examination of epoxy-embedded thick sections reveals vacuolization of many cells in the outer granular layer, consistent with ongoing cytotoxicity (fig. 6).

Biochemical Genetics

Like NLSDI and Refsum disease (RD), SLS is another disorder of nonpolar lipid metabolism that displays an ichthyotic phenotype with additional systemic abnormalities [chapter 1, this vol., table 3, pp. 8–9]. SLS is an autosomal, recessively inherited disorder, affecting 2 embryologically linked tissues of the brain and epidermis, attributable to defective oxidation of long-chain aliphatic alcohols, leading to accumulation of free and esterified, long-chain aliphatic alcohols [105, 106]. A variety of mutations occur in SLS in the *ALDH3A2* gene, encoding the microsomal enzyme FALDH [97, 107].

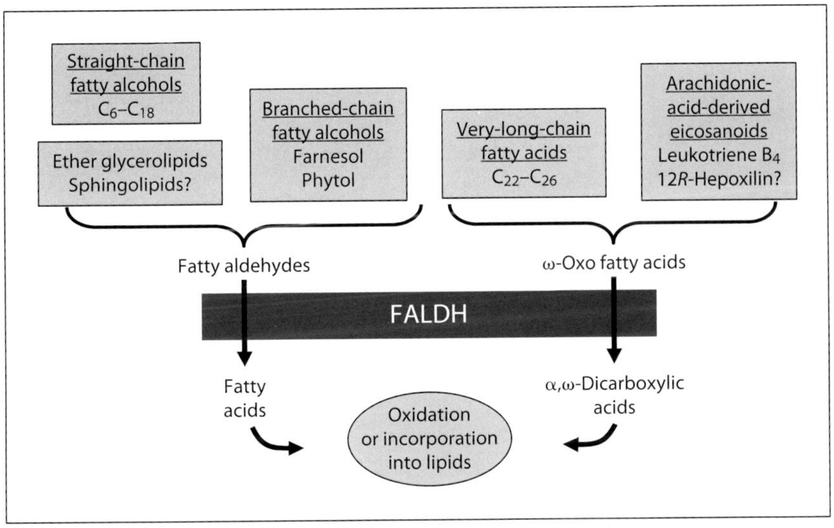

Fig. 8. Lipid metabolites that could account for epidermal structural defects in SLS (courtesy of William Rizzo, MD).

Reduced FALDH activity impairs the oxidation of free fatty alcohols into FFA (fig. 7). However, reduced FFA are not the only biochemical consequence of FALDH deficiency, because a number of other metabolic products can accumulate as a result of FALDH deficiency (fig. 8). These metabolites, in turn, may incorporate into cell membranes, influencing a broad array of cellular pathways, with protean clinical consequences (fig. 8).

Cellular Pathogenesis and Diagnostic Ultrastructure

It is likely that accumulation of one or more lipid metabolites contributes to the SLS cutaneous phenotype (fig. 8). Although biophysical measurements of barrier function in patients have not yet been performed, these lipid abnormality(ies) appear to provoke a permeability barrier abnormality, as demonstrated by increased transdermal lanthanum perfusion, which localizes to extracellular domains of the SC [108] (fig. 9).

The contents of epidermal lamellar bodies are abnormal in SLS (fig. 10) [96, 108]. In addition, the limiting membranes of many individual lamellar bodies exhibit discontinuities, which could account for impaired lamellar body secretion (fig. 10a, b, arrows). Because such membrane discontinuities are not found in other ichthyoses associated with inherited lipid abnormalities, in the authors' opinion, they could represent 'lipotoxicity' from accumulated fatty aldehydes or other bioactive intermediates (fig. 8) [19, 108].

The effects of a disordered lipid metabolism with decreased secretion could explain the observation of both a reduction in lamellar bilayers and prominent, membrane structural abnormalities (fig. 11, 12). With RuO_4 postfixation, it is clear that lamellar/

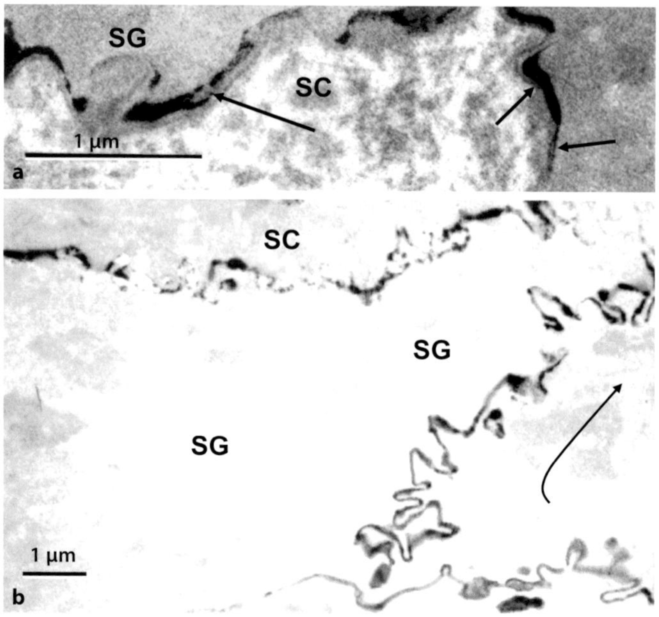

Fig. 9. Lanthanum tracer breaches the SC via the extracellular spaces. This low-molecular-weight, electron-dense tracer reflects the pathway of water movement and is completely excluded from normal SC. The tracer moves outward through the SG (**b**, curved arrow) and remains restricted to SC interstices (**a**, arrows). Thus, the morphological abnormalities in the lamellar body secretory system result in accelerated transcutaneous water loss. OsO_4 postfixation. Magnification bars = 1 µm.

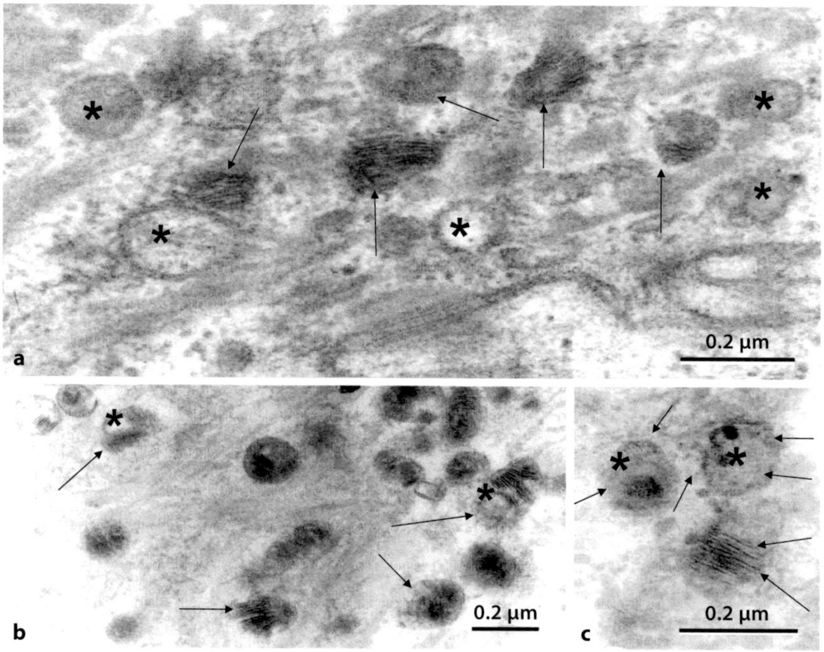

Fig. 10. Abnormal lamellar bodies in SLS. Although the number (density) of lamellar bodies is normal in SLS, many organelles appear empty (asterisks) or display nonlamellar, vesicular contents. Moreover, the limiting membrane of many individual organelles appears disrupted or absent (**a–c**, arrows). OsO_4 postfixation. Magnification bars = 0.2 µm.

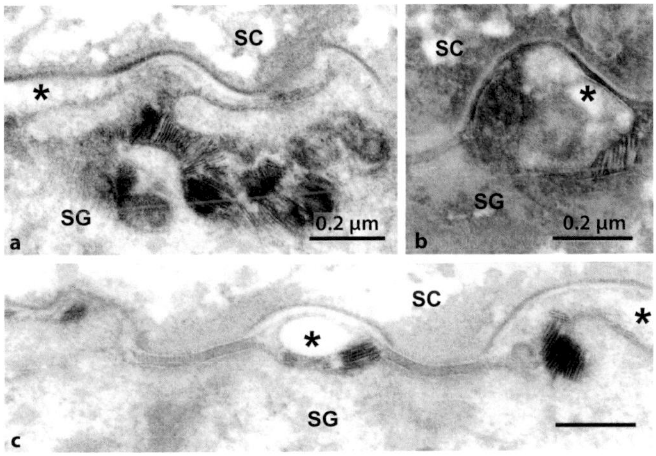

Fig. 11. Decreased lamellar and nonlamellar contents at the SC/SG interface in SLS. Much of it is occupied by vesicular, nonlamellar contents (**a–c**, asterisks) that displace or replace secreted lamellar material. OsO_4 postfixation. Magnification bars = 0.2 µm.

nonlamellar phase separations and a paucity of lamellar bilayers together can account for both the phenotype and the permeability barrier defect in SLS (fig. 13, 14).

While the distinctive features of SLS include the expected abnormality of lamellar/nonlamellar phase separation, as seen in all other lipidoses studied to date (table 3), additional, unexpected and potentially diagnostic findings include: (1) the partial blockade of lamellar body secretion, resulting in entombment of lamellar body contents within corneocytes (fig. 14), a pattern that we otherwise have seen only in ichthyosis associated with inherited protein abnormalities, i.e. epidermolytic ichthyosis and filaggrin-deficient ichthyosis vulgaris, and (2) novel evidence of cytotoxicity, i.e. discontinuities in the limiting membranes of individual lamellar bodies, a finding quite separate from the abnormalities in lamellar body contents (fig. 11). As noted above, these two abnormalities suggest that fatty acid intermediates could provoke profound toxic (i.e. lipotoxic) effects within the cytosol. Notably, this interpretation also fits with one of the proposed pathogenic schemes for ALOX-, NLSDI- and ichthyin-related lipid abnormalities (see fig. 3 and Elias et al. [19]).

2.2.3 Refsum Disease

Keys to Clinical Diagnosis

Late-onset or classic RD (OMIM No. 256500) must be distinguished from infantile RD, an even more global disorder of peroxisomal biogenesis in which peroxisomes fail to form, resulting in loss of function of multiple enzymes. While ichthyosis is not a feature in infantile RD, ichthyosis occurs along with neurological features, including peripheral neuropathy and retinitis pigmentosa, in classic RD. Although severely affected patients can die in childhood, the onset is often insidious, becoming symptomatic only in adolescence, from a disease complex that also includes

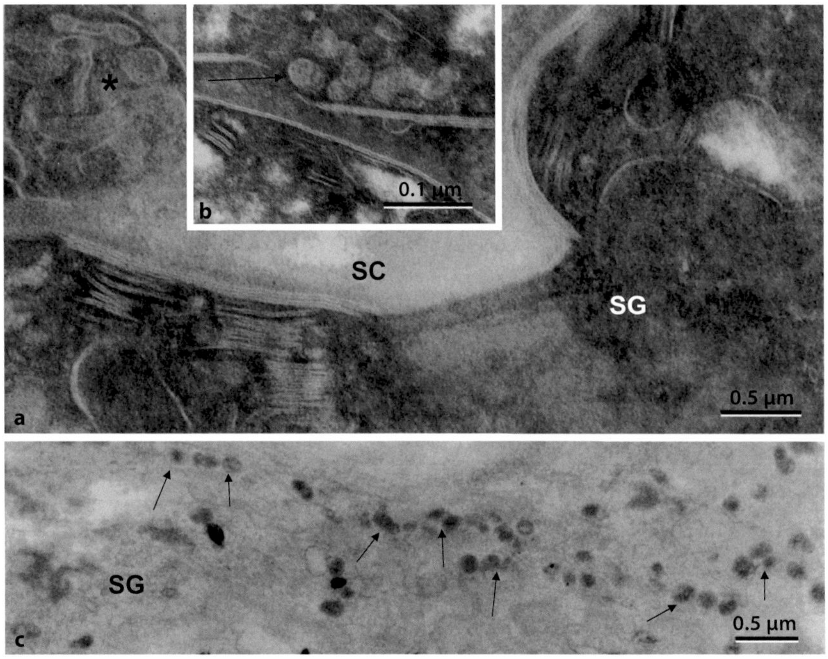

Fig. 12. Abnormal lamellar body secretion results in entombed organelle within corneocytes in SLS. Note concentration of unsecreted lamellar bodies at the periphery of outer SG cells (**c**, arrows). Such unsecreted organelles become entombed in the corneocyte cytosol (**a**, asterisk; **b**, arrow). **a**, **b** RuO_4 postfixation. **c** OsO_4 postfixation. **a**, **c** Magnification bars = 0.5 µm. **b** Magnification bar = 0.1 µm.

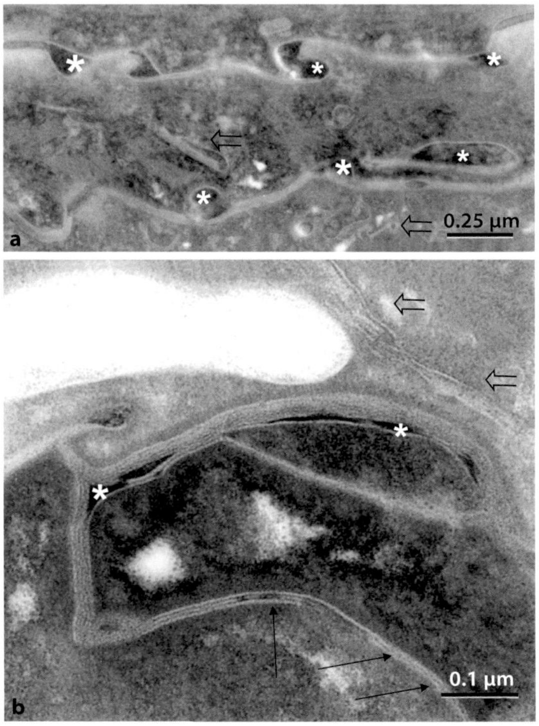

Fig. 13. Decreased lamellar bilayers and lamellar/nonlamellar phase separation in SC interstices. **a**, **b** Entombed lamellar contents in corneocyte cytosol is again evident (open arrows); lamellar domains are interspersed with lacunae filled with nonlamellar material (asterisks). **b** Blockade of secretion (see fig. 4) also results in paucity of lamellar bilayers (arrows). **a**, **b** RuO_4 postfixation. **a** Magnification bar = 0.25 µm. **b** Magnification bar = 0.1 µm.

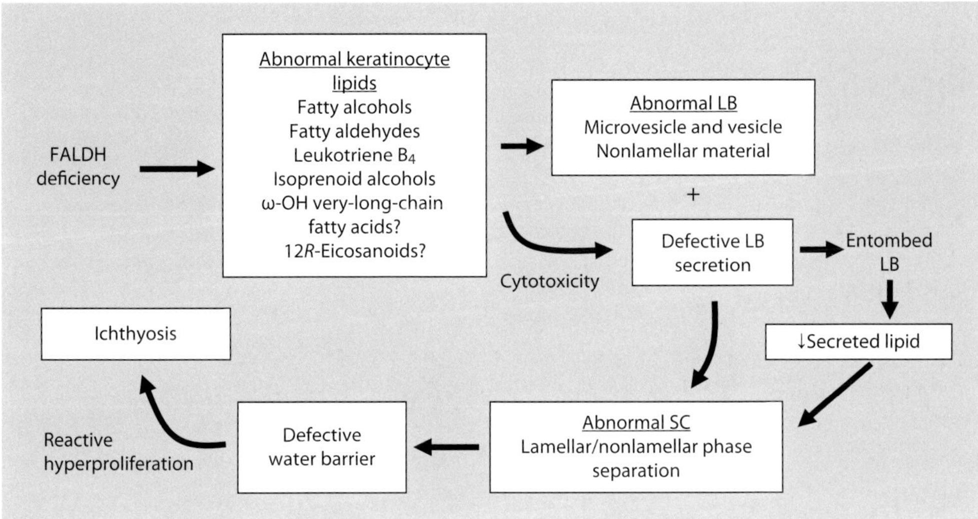

Fig. 14. Cellular pathogenesis of SLS (courtesy of William Rizzo, MD). LB = Lamellar bodies.

deafness, cerebellar ataxia and anosmia [109]. The initial symptom of classic RD is often night blindness, which can progress to severe visual impairment. Mild scaling usually occurs later, during adolescence, or even as late as the fourth or fifth decade [110]. The cutaneous phenotype is similar to ichthyosis vulgaris, with flexural sparing and no erythroderma. Because neurological features do not develop until during or after the second decade of life, the diagnosis is unfortunately often delayed. Earlier recognition (e.g. by ophthalmological examination and/or assessment of plasma phytanic acid levels) would facilitate earlier dietary interventions, which could reduce the severity of the largely irreversible neurological damage. Cardiac arrhythmias may be fatal in RD, but these, as well as other disease symptoms, improve with implementation of a phytol-free diet [95, 109].

Biochemical Genetics

Classic RD is a rare, autosomal, recessively inherited disorder of peroxisome metabolism due to a defect in the initial step in the β-oxidation of phytanic acid, a C_{16} saturated fatty acid with 4 methyl side groups (at the C3, 7, 11 and 15 positions) [95, 109]. In RD, the peroxisomal β-oxidation of phytanic acid is blocked by the presence of the methyl group at the 3-position. Yet, accumulation of phytanic acid, though characteristic of RD, is not pathognomonic, since elevated plasma phytanic acid levels occur in other peroxisomal disorders, including global peroxisomal deficiencies, such as infantile RD and in rhizomelic chondrodysplasia punctata (see below) [95]. Nonetheless, within an appropriate clinical setting, the biochemical diagnosis of RD can be made by finding elevated phytanic acid levels in plasma. Multisystem accumulation of

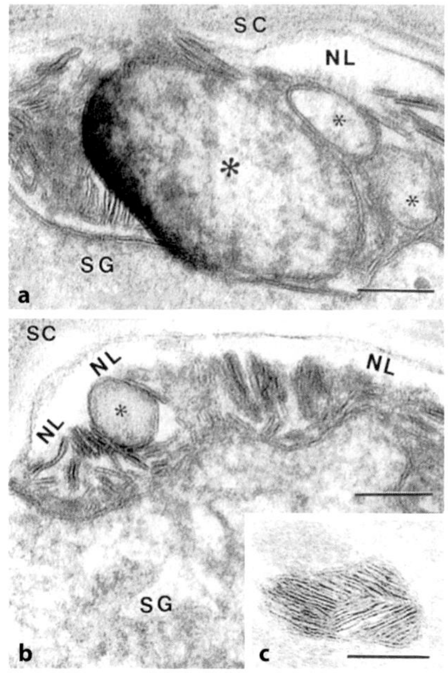

Fig. 15. Abnormalities in the lamellar body secretory system in RD. **a, b** Coalescence of neutral-lipid (NL) droplets (asterisks). **c** Distribution of individual lamellar bodies. Magnification bars = 0.1 µm.

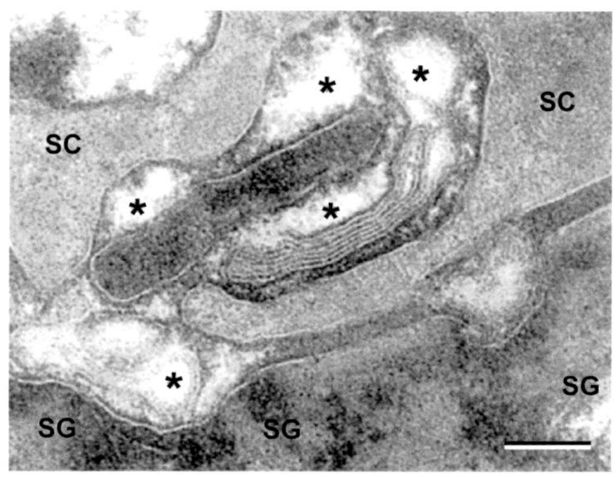

Fig. 16. Disruption of secreted lamellar body contents by nonlamellar material in RD (asterisks). Magnification bar = 0.1 µm.

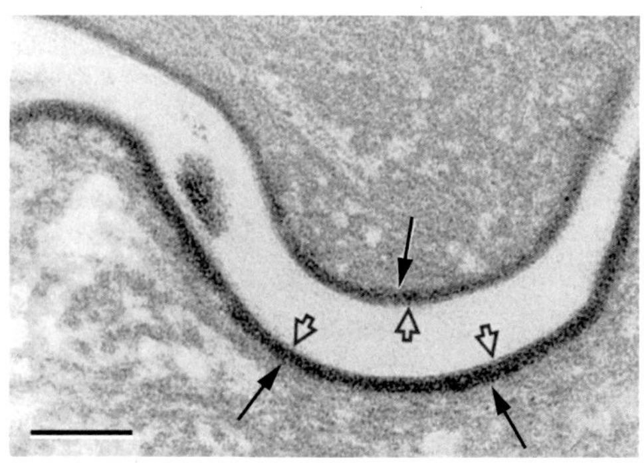

Fig. 17. Loss of corneocyte lipid envelope in RD (open arrows). Magnification bar = 0.1 µm.

phytols, predominantly phytanic acid, occurs at up to millimolar concentrations, and defective phytanic acid oxidation can be demonstrated in cultured fibroblasts [95].

While mutations in the gene encoding phytanoyl coenzyme A hydroxylase *(PAHX, PHYH)* occur in up to 80% of classic RD patients [109], some patients instead have mutations in the peroxin 7 receptor (*PEX7*) [111]. *PEX7* mutations also underlie a severer phenotype, rhizomelic chondrodysplasia punctata (OMIM No. 21508), in which severe skeletal defects predominate [111, 112]. Although a mild ichthyosis reportedly occurs in about one third of patients with rhizomelic chondrodysplasia punctata [113], it is not well described.

Pathology and Pathogenesis

It has been proposed that the disease complex in RD can be explained in part by the high affinity of phytanic acid for the retinoid X receptor and/or PPAR-α [112, 114]. Although purely speculative, the symptoms of RD mimic several features of hypervitaminosis A, which also includes visual, neurological and desquamatory abnormalities. However, phytanic acid can have other effects. It induces apoptosis in cardiac and neuronal cells, and it mobilizes Ca^{2+} from mitochondrial stores [95]. Moreover, other lipotoxic pathomechanisms, similar to those proposed for NLSDI and SLS, could also be operative (fig. 3). The relative role of these divergent mechanisms in disease pathogenesis remains unknown.

Ultrastructure and Possible Pathogenesis

The following abnormalities were noted in 2 unrelated patients with RD by Blanchet-Bardon et al. [110]: (1) epidermal hyperplasia; (2) an increased number of cornified cell layers (30–40 layers); (3) presence of cells (perhaps melanocytes) with large, oil-red-O-positive cytoplasmic vacuoles, within the basal cell layer, and (4) reduction of the granular layer to a single layer. However, F-type keratohyalin granules and lamellar body number (density) and secretion appeared to be normal.

We recently examined biopsies from 2 unrelated, genotyped RD patients. Although lamellar body density was normal, the shape of individual organelles was often distorted (fig. 15c illustrates a 'pyramidal' shape), and the organelles also often contained interspersed nonlamellar material. This amorphous material subsequently appears as nonlamellar domains at the SG/SC interface (fig. 15a, b), often coalescing into large droplets that displace secreted lamellae (fig. 15a and 16, asterisks). The most striking ultrastructural observation is the partial detachment or complete absence of the corneocyte lipid envelope in RD (fig. 17, open arrows). This intriguing observation, however, needs to be confirmed by lipid biochemistry (i.e. are bound ω-hydroxyceramides reduced or absent?). In summary, RD represents another disease with abnormal lamellar/nonlamellar phase separation, but with distinctive abnormalities both in the lamellar body secretory system and in the corneocyte lipid envelope. The abnormal SC membranes with phase separation could be due to the substitution of branched-chain fatty acids for unbranched species, and a failure of these fatty acids to incorporate into lamellar structures. Similarly, branched-chain FA may be unable to serve as substrates for one of the enzymes that lead to formation of ω-OH-ceramides. Thus, the cutaneous phenotype in RD is consistent with bulk effects of phytanic acid-derived FA on SC structure and function.

2.3. Multisystem Diseases of Cholesterol Metabolism

2.3.1 Conradi-Hünermann-Happle Syndrome (Chondrodysplasia Punctata) and Congenital Hemidysplasia with Ichthyosiform Erythroderma and Limb Defects

Clinical Features

The cutaneous features in Conradi-Hünermann-Happle syndrome (CHH) or X-linked dominant chondrodysplasia punctata type 2 (OMIM No. 302960) are most striking in the neonate. Linear bands of scaling or follicular spikes (with calcium seen in follicles histologically) occur in a morphogenic pattern (i.e. along the lines of Blaschko), accompanied by a generalized erythroderma. Involved skin sites are presumed to conform to regions in which the mutant X chromosome remains the active X chromosome [115, 116]. The cutaneous features of CHH slowly resolve after infancy, leaving atrophy (follicular atrophoderma), alopecia and occasionally mild ichthyosis on the extremities [116]. Chondrodysplasia punctata denotes an abnormality in bone formation, visualized radiographically as stippled epiphyses, and occurs not only in CHH, but also in congenital hemidysplasia with ichthyosiform erythroderma and limb defects (CHILD syndrome; see below) and in other inherited peroxisomal disorders. Disease severity in chondrodysplasia punctata is dependent upon both the specific mutation and the extent to which the mutant X chromosome remains 'active' in bone and other affected tissues [117–120]. The gradual resolution of the ichthyosiform phenotype presumably reflects a dilution of skin effects due to diminished viability of keratinocytes which bear an active mutant X chromosome [99].

The cutaneous phenotype in CHILD syndrome (OMIM No. 308050) is unique and differs in its distribution from CHH, i.e. it is strictly limited to one side of the body and can involve nails and hair [121, 122]. Skeletal defects and internal organ involvement also are restricted to the involved side. Interestingly, the right side is more commonly affected, probably because of lethality from cardiac involvement with left-sided disease expression. Skin lesions are prominent, circumscribed plaques, surrounded by wax-like scales, which may partially resolve, as in CHH. Yet, flexures typically remain involved, and in contrast to CHH, the atrophoderma does not resolve [123]. In addition to these features, neonatal CHH syndrome biopsies can display Ca^{2+} in hair follicles [24]. The limited skin and skeletal distribution of CHILD syndrome likely also represents the extent to which the mutant X chromosome remains active. It should be noted, however, that our ultrastructural studies show that the 'uninvolved side' of

CHILD syndrome is not completely uninvolved, i.e. it displays distinctive abnormalities in the lamellar body secretory system (see below).

Biochemical Genetics

Both of these multisystem syndromes, i.e. CHH and CHILD syndrome, are caused by mutations in genes encoding enzymes of the distal (i.e. postsqualene) cholesterol biosynthetic pathway. CHH is usually caused by mutations in the emopamil-binding protein gene that encodes 3β-hydroxysterol-Δ^8,Δ^7-isomerase, which catalyzes the conversion of 8(9)-cholestenol to lathosterol [117, 124, 125]. Loss of functions in this enzyme results in diagnostic elevations of the sterol precursors, 8-dehydrocholesterol and 8(9)-cholesterol in serum [121]. Mutations in *NSDHL*, which encodes a member of the enzyme complex that removes the C_4 methyl group in the next-most proximal step in the sterol synthetic pathway, which catalyzes the conversion of lanosterol to lathosterol, underlie CHILD syndrome. However, CHILD syndrome can also be caused by mutations in emopamil-binding protein gene [121, 126]. Given the close approximation of the sites of metabolic blockade and the striking phenotypic similarities, the presence of some phenotypic overlap is not surprising (reviewed in Kelley and Herman [126]).

While a scaling phenotype does not occur in Smith-Lemli-Opitz syndrome (OMIM No. 270400), caused by 7-dehydrocholesterol reductase deficiency, ichthyosis does develop in hairless mice treated with the 7-dehydrocholesterol inhibitor AY9944 [127]. Inhibitor-induced blockade of the Δ^{24}-reductase, which converts desmosterol to cholesterol, by either triparanol or 20,25-diazocholesterol, also provokes ichthyosis in both rodent models and in humans [127, 128]. It is likely, therefore, that 7-dehydrocholesterol, but not desmosterol, can partially substitute for cholesterol in the formation of SC lamellar membranes. Cholesterol is one of the key lipids (with ceramides and FFA) that are required to form mature lamellar membranes, and such cholesterol-deficient membranes provide a suboptimal barrier (reviewed in Feingold [129]). Thus, an additional pathomechanism could also be operative in CHILD and CHH syndromes, i.e. substitution of distal sterol precursors (7-dehydrocholesterol/zymosterol) for cholesterol could result in defective lamellar membranes.

Pathology and Cellular Pathogenesis

Although the pathophysiological basis for the ichthyosiform phenotype is not yet known, the pathogenesis of CHH and CHILD syndromes is likely to be similar to that of other ichthyoses attributable to inborn errors of lipid metabolism. The multisystem malformations that result from disorders of postsqualene sterologenesis have been attributed variously to: (1) deficiency of bulk cholesterol in cell membranes with resulting functional alterations; (2) toxic effects of accumulated sterol precursors, and/or (3) developmental effects of altered hedgehog pathway signaling (its proteins are tethered onto cell membranes via a cholesterol moiety [130]).

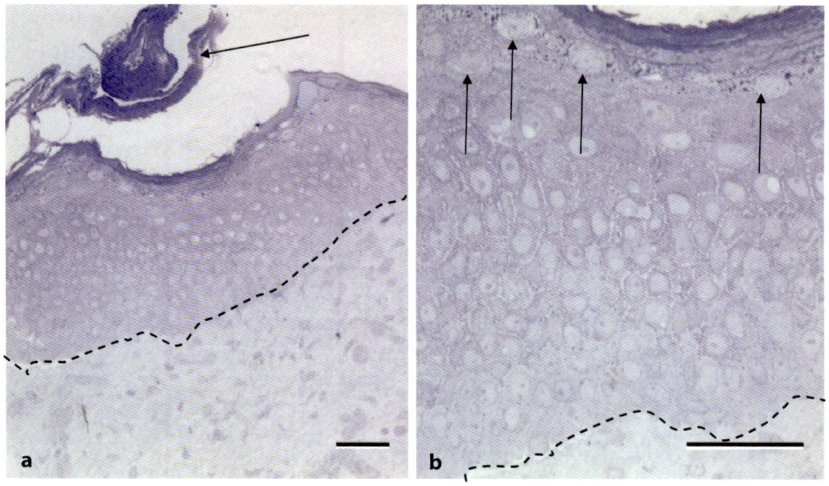

Fig. 18. Histopathology of CHH. The epidermis displays striking epidermal hyperplasia, with presence of a vacuolated granular layer (**b**, arrows) and a loosely coherent SC (**a**, long arrow). Magnification bars = 5 µm.

Prior to the identification of primary sterologenesis defects in CHH and CHILD syndromes, these disorders were thought to be disorders of peroxisomal biogenesis (see above). Deficient peroxisomal function has been described in cultured fibroblasts from both CHH and CHILD patients [114, 131–134], as well as in the murine homologue, the 'bare patches' mouse [99], which displays transient cutaneous clinical and morphological defects, similar to CHH, but now attributed to *Nsdhl* mutations [99, 135] (as underlie CHILD syndrome). Pertinently, the clinical phenotypes of both the postsqualene sterologenesis and the peroxisome biogenesis disorders bear certain striking resemblances [135], including skeletal defects (chondrodysplasia punctata), CNS and hepatic involvement, as well as ichthyosis. The partial localization of all these postsqualene enzymes within peroxisomes could explain such a phenotypic overlap (cited in Emami et al. [99]).

Diagnostic Ultrastructure

Conradi-Hünermann-Happle Syndrome. While light microscopy reveals prominent epidermal hyperplasia and a vacuolated granular layer (fig. 18), low-magnification electron micrographs reveal further, substantial changes in the SG, including keratin filament disorganization in CHH (fig. 19).

In CHH, both the density of lamellar bodies and lamellar body secretion appear normal (fig. 19), but newly secreted material fails to disburse at the SG/SC interface (fig. 20 and 21). Lamellar body contents, however, are abnormal, displaying vesicular inclusions (fig. 20b, inset), as found in NLSDI, SLS and RD. Furthermore, these electron-lucent vesicles persist as discrete spheres after secretion at the SG/SC interface

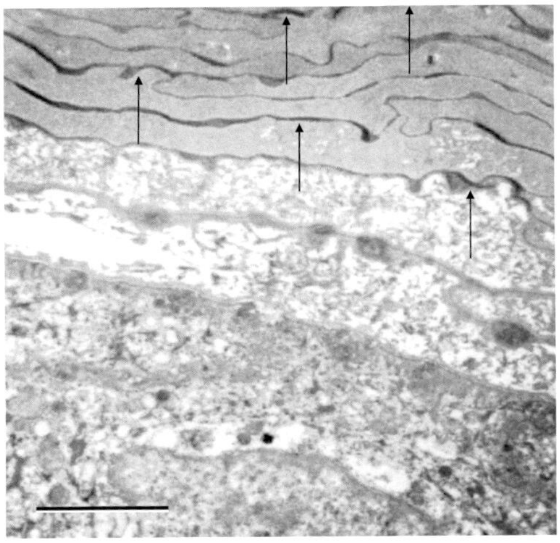

Fig. 19. Low magnification ultrastructure of CHH. Lamellar body secretion appears to be unimpaired, but note that unprocessed, secreted material persists high into the SC (arrows). OsO_4 postfixation. Magnification bar = 0.5 µm.

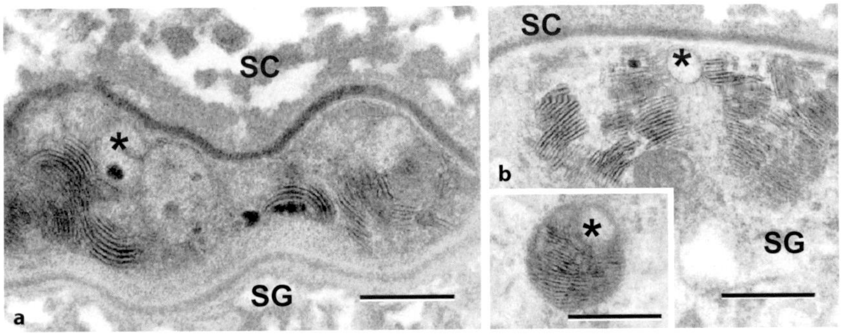

Fig. 20. Abnormal lamellar body contents and postsecretory dispersion in CHH (asterisks). Magnification bars = 0.5 µm.

(fig. 21b). Importantly, maturation of lamellar bilayers is delayed (fig. 19 and 21b), and membranes are displaced by extensive areas of lamellar/nonlamellar phase separation [99]. In contrast to these abnormalities in the lamellar body secretory system, cornified envelopes, the corneocyte lipid envelope and corneodesmosomes all appear normal in CHH.

CHILD Syndrome. The ultrastructural morphology of clinically affected skin sites in CHILD syndrome is also dramatically abnormal, potentially comprising a diagnostic pattern. Lamellar bodies appear to be formed normally but display almost no internal lamellae (fig. 22b). These organelles fuse into multivesicular bodies, which are then largely (but incompletely) secreted (fig. 22a, b). The SC displays a huge expansion of the extracellular matrix, which is filled with interspersed lamellar and nonlamellar material (fig. 23). Yet, the corneocyte envelope and the corneocyte lipid envelope appear normal (fig. 20). While it is possible that

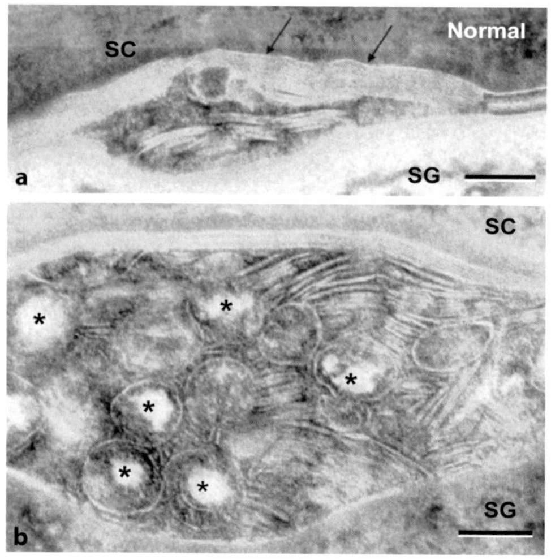

Fig. 21. Abnormal secreted lamellar body contents and delayed processing into mature lamellar bilayers in CHH. Arrows = normal lamellar bilayers; asterisks = 'empty' lamellar body contents. Magnification bars = 0.5 μm.

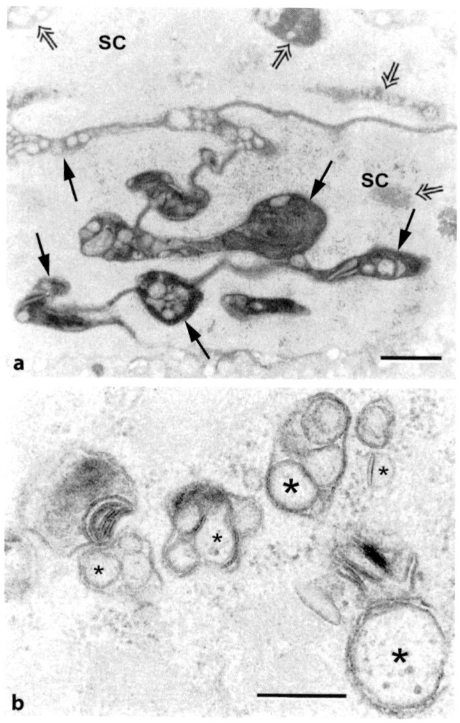

Fig. 22. Abnormal lamellar body structure and aberrant secretion in CHILD syndrome. Lamellar bodies, with minimal recognizable contents, fuse with one another, forming multivesicular organelles (**b**). Abnormal contents are secreted prematurely, and persist within the SC interstices. Arrows = premature secretion; open arrows = entombed lamellar bodies; asterisks = coalescence of unsecreted lamellar bodies.
a Magnification bar = 0.05 μm. **b** Magnification bar = 0.25 μm.

this extracellular abnormality could reflect inspissated topical emollients, similar features were found at all levels of the SC, and in tissue samples from 2 different patients. These abnormalities are sufficiently distinctive to be potentially diagnostic of CHILD syndrome. As noted above, lesser abnormalities in the lamellar body

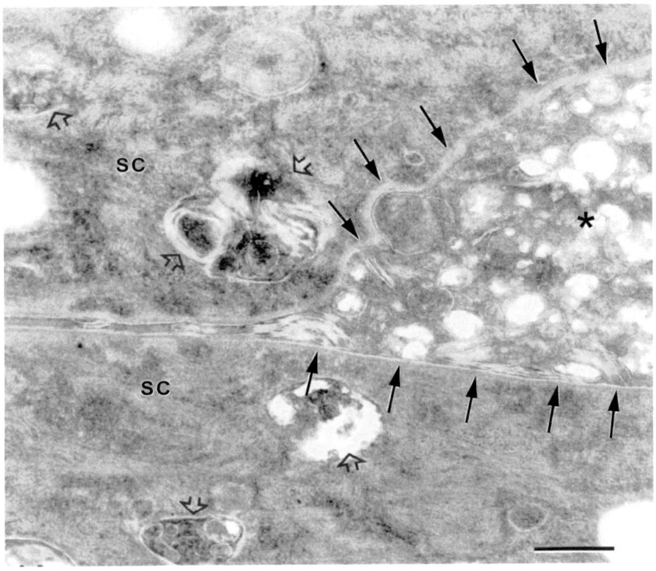

Fig. 23. Expansion and disorganization of the SC interstices in CHILD syndrome (asterisk). Note the lack of lamellar bilayers, but preservation of the corneocyte lipid envelope (arrows). Entombed lamellar body contents (open arrows) indicates partial failure of secretion. Magnification bar = 0.2 µm.

secretory system and lamellar bilayers are also evident in the 'uninvolved' skin of CHILD syndrome.

2.3.2 Recessive X-Linked Ichthyosis

Clinical Features

The ichthyosiform phenotype of RXLI (OMIM No. 308100) is noted soon after birth, typically as generalized peeling or exaggerated neonatal desquamation, but in some instances RXLI may present with a collodion membrane. After the neonatal period, fine scaling is present on the trunk and extremities. In older boys and men, scales often become coarser and darker over time. While scaling is generalized, it typically spares the antecubital and popliteal fossae. The midface is also spared, but the lateral face may be involved, and the neck is almost always involved. Axillae are also frequently involved, while the palms and soles are spared. While the clinical features are quite similar to ichthyosis vulgaris, the browner color of the scale and the more 'centripetal' distribution with involvement of the neck and axillary flexures, but sparing of the palms/soles usually suggest the clinical diagnosis of RXLI. Nevertheless, there is sufficient phenotypic overlap to require further studies to reliably distinguish between these two disorders. Indeed, both of these disorders are relatively common (RXLI occurs from 1/2,000 to 1/6,000 males, and filaggrin mutations in a ratio of 1:10), and their concurrence could result in a severer clinical phenotype [136]. Routine histopathology is unremarkable in RXLI, showing moderate hyperkeratosis with mild acanthosis and preservation of the granular cell layer. Measurement of substrate accumulation in skin (cholesterol sulfate) or blood (cholesterol sulfate or other sulfated steroid hormones) is diagnostic, as is an assay of steroid sulfatase (SSase) activity in cultured fibroblasts or leukocytes [137, 138]. Because most RXLI cases arise from deletion of the *STS* gene, fluorescence in situ hybridization testing for this gene is the most commonly employed clinical test, but this assay can yield false-negative results in individuals who have point mutations (probably <10% of RXLI). Serum lipoprotein electrophoresis is also diagnostic, demonstrating more rapid mobility of the low-density lipoprotein (LDL; β) and pre-LDL (pre-β) fractions due to an increased sulfated sterol content [137, 139].

RXLI is a systemic, albeit usually mild, disorder. Placental sulfatase deficiency syndrome, occurring in pregnancies of RXLI fetuses, can manifest as failure of labor to either initiate or to progress, failed cervical softening and a poor response to pitocin, and can be detected by extremely low maternal urinary and blood estriol levels [140–142]. Since estriol levels are part of the so-called triple screen test employed to detect pregnancies at risk for chromosomal defects, many RXLI fetuses are now detected in this manner [143, 144]. In contrast to previous estimates, the incidence of cryptorchidism (testicular maldescent) does not appear to exceed 5%. Testicular cancer has been reported in a few RXLI patients with normally descended testes [145]; however, in the absence of follow-up reports, it is difficult to determine if this is a chance association. Small, comma-shaped corneal opacities develop in the posterior capsule of Descemet's membrane in approximately 50% of adult RXLI patients, but these are often not present in children. These opacities are entirely asymptomatic, though diagnostic when present; however, their absence does not exclude the diagnosis of RXLI. Female carriers do not exhibit ichthyosis or other clinical signs, though they too may exhibit asymptomatic corneal opacities. Finally, some RXLI patients can exhibit cognitive behavior abnormalities, presumably due to deletion of contiguous genes.

When males present with generalized ichthyosis in the setting of multisystem disease, the possibility for RXLI as part of a contiguous gene syndrome should be considered. Because RXLI results from deletion of the *STS* gene, additional neighboring genes on the distal tip of the short arm of the X chromosome can also be affected. Kallman's syndrome, which occurs in about 1/10,000 males, displays anosmia, hypogonadism, variable mental retardation, ichthyosis and a number of other findings, represents one such contiguous gene syndrome (see below).

Biochemical Genetics

RXLI almost only affects males, who display primarily loss-of-function mutations in the gene encoding the microsomal enzyme SSase [146, 147], but rarely, homozygous females have been noted. *SSase* is located on the distal tip of the short arm of the X chromosome [140, 148–151]; deletions in *SSase* [152–156] can provoke ichthyosiform skin changes alone, or a syndromic ichthyosis with extracutaneous organ system involvement, if contiguous genes are also deleted (contiguous gene syndromes) [157–159]. SSase is a classic microsomal enzyme that further localizes to coated pits in the plasma membrane [160, 161], where it hydrolyzes the 3β-sulfate esters from both cholesterol sulfate (CSO_4) and a large family of sulfated steroid hormones (fig. 24).

While SSase activity is normally low in the basal and spinous layers of the epidermis, it increases in the outer epidermis, peaking in the granular layer (approx. 5% of total lipid) [162], and persisting into the SC (fig. 25). In cytochemical studies, SSase activity localizes not only within the cytosol (i.e. microsomes), but also within lamellar bodies and within the interstices of the lower SC following lamellar body secretion [94]. Thus, SSase, like other lipid hydrolases that are involved in the extracellular processing of secreted polar lipids, utilizes the lamellar body secretory system to reach sites where it participates in the regulation of permeability barrier homeostasis and desquamation [87].

The 'Cholesterol Sulfate Cycle' and Its Regulatory Significance

Cholesterol sulfotransferase (SULT2B1b) activity generates cholesterol sulfate predominately in the lower nucleated cell layers of the epidermis, while in contrast SSase peaks in the outer epidermis. Hence, Epstein et al. [163] proposed that an 'epidermal cholesterol sulfate cycle' exists in the epidermis in which cholesterol is first sulfated in the lower epidermis (fig. 25 and 26) and then desulfated back to cholesterol in the outer epidermal nucleated layers. Thus, the epidermal content of cholesterol sulfate increases from 1 to 5% of total lipid as cells move from the basal to the granular layer and then declines again to 1% as corneocytes move from the inner to the outer SC [164, 165] (fig. 25). Disruption of this cholesterol sulfate cycle accounts for both the abnormal desquamation and the permeability barrier abnormality in RXLI (see below).

Sulfation of cholesterol by SULT2B1b is intimately linked to epidermal differentiation [165–167], including normal cornification [168–170]. This relationship is shown convincingly by the observation that cholesterol sulfate levels are several orders of magnitude higher in keratinizing than in mucosal epithelia [167]. Conversely, reversal of keratinization, through induction of mucous metaplasia in keratinizing epithelia (e.g. by application of exogenous retinoids) dramatically reduces tissue cholesterol sulfate levels [168, 171]. Moreover, both SULT2B1b expression and cholesterol sulfate levels increase late in epidermal development in utero [172, 173], in parallel with the formation of a functionally competent SC [174]. Finally, retinoic acid, which inhibits differentiation, also inhibits SULT2B1b expression, PPAR-δ and liver X receptor activators, which stimulate differentiation and also increase SULT2B1b expression [175].

Cholesterol sulfate is itself a potent transcriptional regulator in both cutaneous and extracutaneous tissues [176, 177], stimulating epidermal differentiation by at least 2 related mechanisms (fig. 25 and 27). First, it activates the η-isoform of protein kinase C [178–180], which in turn stimulates the phosphorylation of differentiation-linked proteins, assessed as increased cornified envelope formation [181]. Second, cholesterol sulfate is a transcriptional regulator of proteins involved in cornified

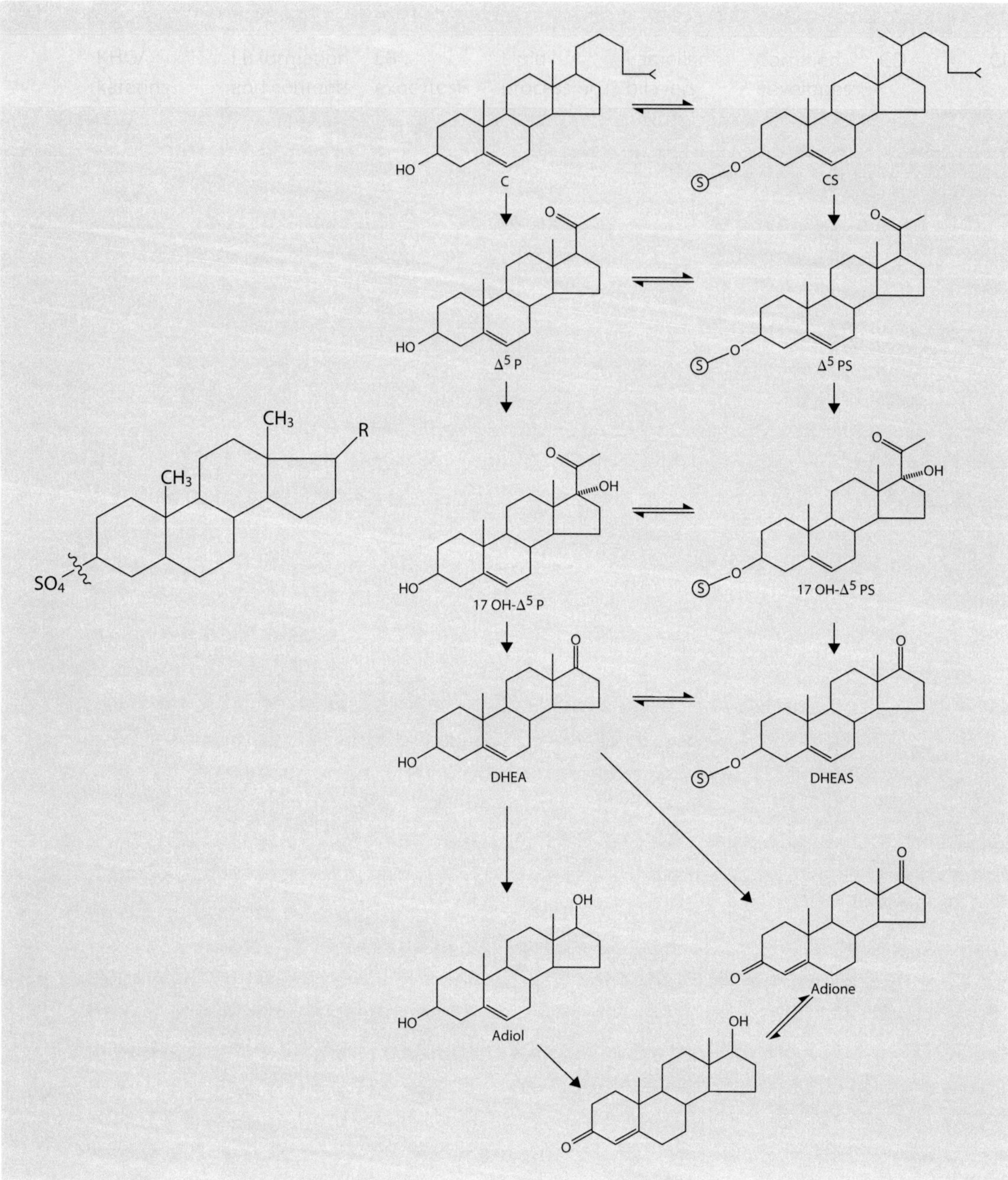

Fig. 24. SSase desulfates cholesterol sulfate and other sulfated steroid hormones.

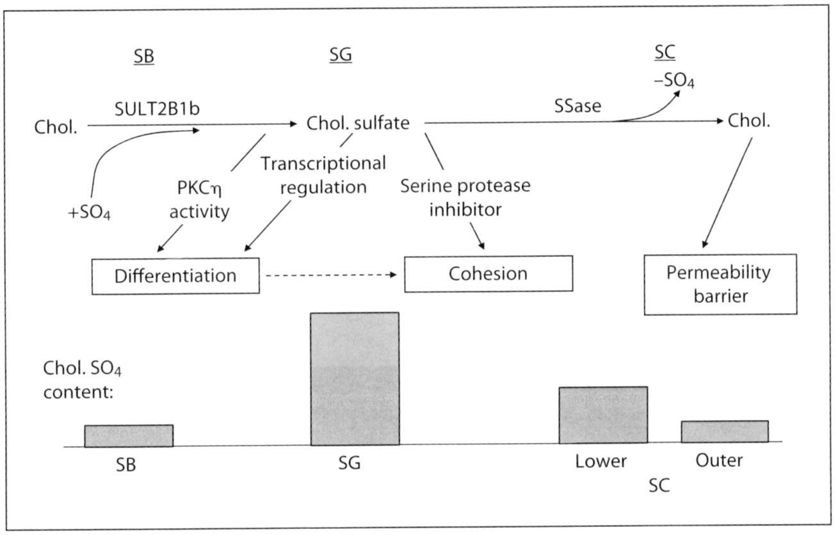

Fig. 25. Multiple epidermal functions impacted by cholesterol sulfate (modified from Elias et al. [94]). SB = Stratum basale; chol. = cholesterol; PKC = protein kinase C.

Fig. 26. Epidermal cholesterol sulfate cycle (modified from Epstein et al. [163]). LXR = Liver X receptor.

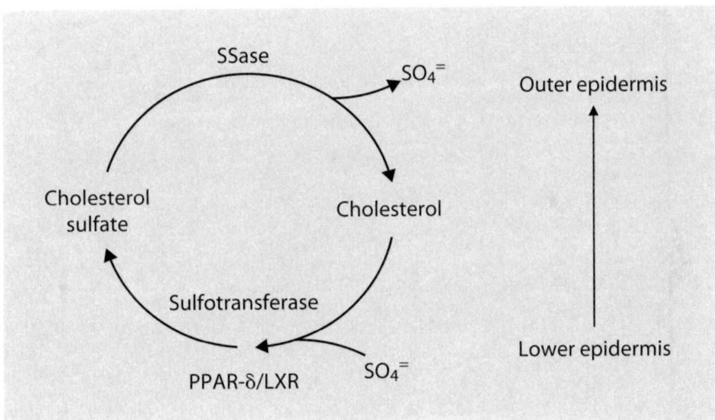

envelope formation, such as TGM-1 and involucrin, operating through an adaptor-protein (AP)-1-binding site in the promoter region [182, 183]. It is likely that these two mechanisms are linked, because protein kinase C activation by cholesterol sulfate could phosphorylate AP-1, leading to enhanced transcriptional regulation of TGM-1 and involucrin (fig. 27). Together, these observations provide a molecular explanation for the multiple biological consequences of an altered cholesterol sulfate cycle.

Pathology and Pathogenesis

As a result of enzyme deficiency in RXLI, cholesterol sulfate accumulates in the epidermis [137, 162, 184], in erythrocyte cell membranes [137, 138] and in both the LDL

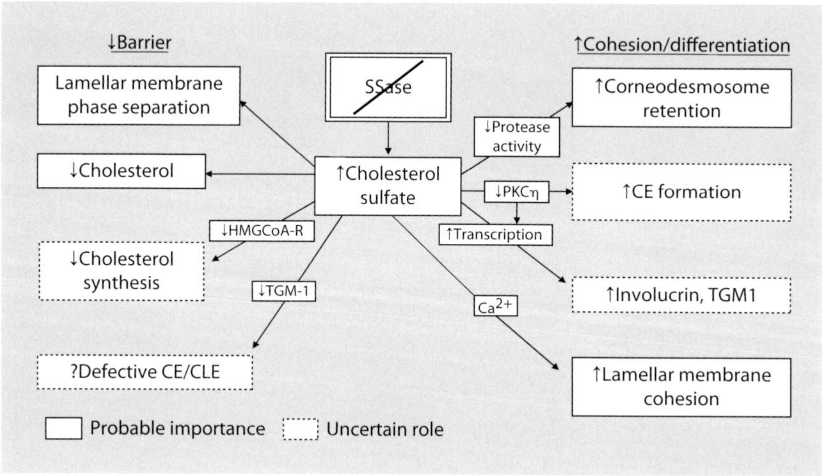

Fig. 27. Potential pathogenetic mechanisms in RXLI (modified from Elias et al. [94]). CE = Cornified envelope; CLE = corneocyte lipid envelope; PKC = protein kinase C; HMGCoA-R = hydroxymethylglutaryl coenzyme A reductase; TGM1 = transglutaminase 1.

(β-lipoprotein) and pre-LDL fractions of plasma [137], but cholesterol sulfate levels in the epidermis are an order of magnitude higher than levels in blood [137, 138], likely explaining the prominence of skin versus other organ involvement in RXLI [185]. As noted above, cholesterol sulfate levels normally decline to about 1% of lipid mass in the outer SC, through ongoing hydrolysis during SC transit [164, 186] (fig. 25). In contrast, the SC in RXLI typically contains 10–12% cholesterol sulfate (by dry weight) [185]. Although SSase is secreted from lamellar bodies (like other barrier lipid precursors), cholesterol sulfate is not concentrated in lamellar bodies [94, 187]. Its mode of delivery to the SC interstices instead is likely explained by its extreme amphiphilicity, allowing it to diffuse readily across cell membranes [188], i.e. in the absence of a lipid milieu within corneocytes, cholesterol sulfate likely partitions preferentially into the highly hydrophobic, extracellular domains of the SC.

Basis for the Permeability Barrier Abnormality in Recessive X-Linked Ichthyosis

Patients with RXLI display a minimal, but significant basal barrier abnormality [189, 190], with a pronounced delay in recovery kinetics following acute perturbations [191], suggesting that excess cholesterol sulfate destabilizes permeability barrier homeostasis (fig. 28). In support of this hypothesis, excess cholesterol sulfate forms nonlamellar domains in model lipid mixtures and in RXLI scale [92, 93]. Yet, the barrier abnormality could also be due in part to the decreased cholesterol content of the SC in RXLI (reduced by approx. 50%) [185]. A comparable decrease in cholesterol produces a barrier abnormality in conjunction with the formation of abnormal extracellular lamellar membranes in experimental animals [192]. Thus, to

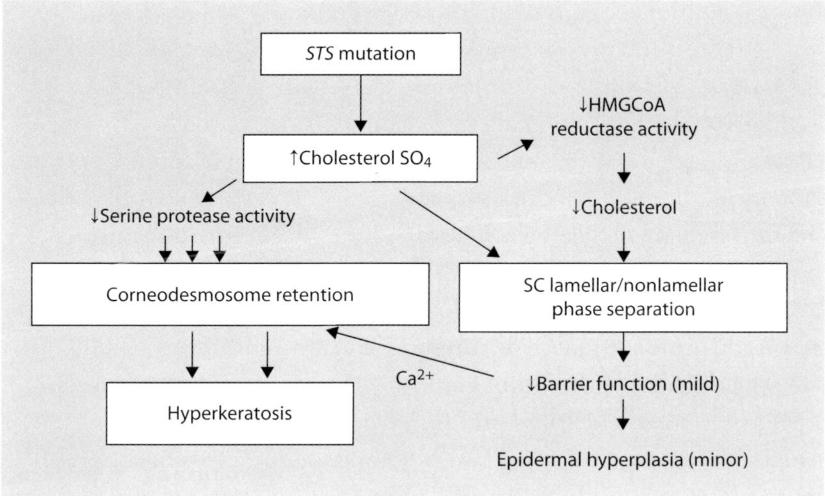

Fig. 28. Pathogenesis of X-linked ichthyosis. HMGCoA = Hydroxymethylglutaryl coenzyme A.

varying degrees, the decrease in cholesterol in RXLI could be due to either reduced generation of cholesterol from cholesterol sulfate due to the enzyme deficiency [191, 193] and/or to cholesterol-sulfate-mediated inhibition of hydroxymethylglutaryl coenzyme A reductase, the rate-limiting enzyme of cholesterol synthesis [193] (fig. 28). In summary, the dominant mechanisms that account for the barrier abnormality in RXLI appear to be: (1) lamellar/nonlamellar phase separation due to excess cholesterol sulfate and (2) reduced cholesterol content of the SC lamellar membranes [94].

Mechanisms Accounting for Abnormal Desquamation in Recessive X-Linked Ichthyosis
Kinetic studies have demonstrated that the hyperkeratosis in RXLI reflects delayed desquamation [194]. The basis for this classic retention type of ichthyosis is persistence of corneodesmosomes at all levels of the SC (fig. 28 and 29). Two key serine proteases, kallikrein 7 (SC chymotryptic enzyme) and kallikrein 5 (SC tryptic enzyme) are primary mediators of corneodesmosome degradation in vitro [195]. Cholesterol sulfate appears to increase SC retention through the known ability of this lipid to function as a serine protease inhibitor [94, 196, 197] (fig. 30). Moreover, while the acidic pH of the SC inhibits the activities of SC chymotryptic enzyme and SC tryptic enzyme [198–200], the pH of the SC in RXLI is even more acidic than normal [201]. Hence, serine protease activity is reduced dramatically in RXLI (fig. 30) [94].

The SC in RXLI demonstrates abundant Ca^{2+} in extracellular domains, which preferentially localizes along the external faces of opposing corneodesmosomes (fig. 31b) [94]. Thus, the delayed degradation of corneodesmosomes in RXLI could be due in part to leakage of Ca^{2+} into the lower SC (due to the barrier defect), with formation of

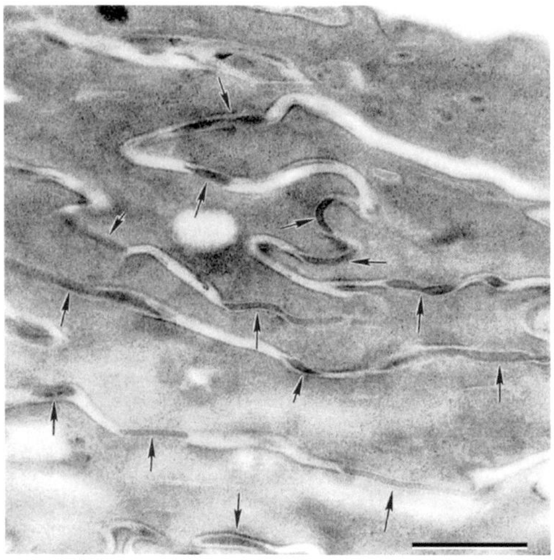

Fig. 29. Persistence of corneodesmosomes (arrows) at all levels of the SC in RXLI. Magnification bar = 0.5 μm.

Ca^{2+} bridges between adjacent corneodesmosomes [94]. Ca^{2+}, if present in sufficient quantities, can stabilize highly anionic SO_4 groups (from persistent cholesterol sulfate) on lamellar bilayers [163]. Indeed, CSO_4-containing liposomes aggregate avidly in the presence of Ca^{2+} [202, 203].

Diagnostic Ultrastructure

Lamellar body density and contents appear normal in RXLI, as is the morphology of individual corneodesmosomes. The key diagnostic features on electron microscopy are: (1) the persistence of 'pristine' corneodesmosomes, i.e. little evidence of proteolysis, high into the SC (fig. 29), and (2) the presence of frequent, focal sites of electron-dense, nonlamellar material, which disrupts the organization of the extracellular lamellae [94, 191] (fig. 31a). The combination of marked corneodesmosome retention with lamellar/nonlamellar phase separation is diagnostic of RXLI.

2.4. Multisystem Diseases of Sphingolipid Metabolism

2.4.1 Gaucher Disease

Clinical Features and Biochemical Genetics

Three recognized variants of GD (type 1: OMIM No. 230800, type 2: No. 230900, type 3: No. 231000) are all caused by recessive mutations in the autosomal gene encoding β-glucocerebrosidase, which removes the glucose moiety from glucosylceramides, generating free ceramides [204]. Yet, an ichthyosiform phenotype is only observed in the severest, the type 2 (acute neuronopathic) form of GD [98, 205]. Infants with type 2 GD can present with a collodion baby phenotype at birth in conjunction with other

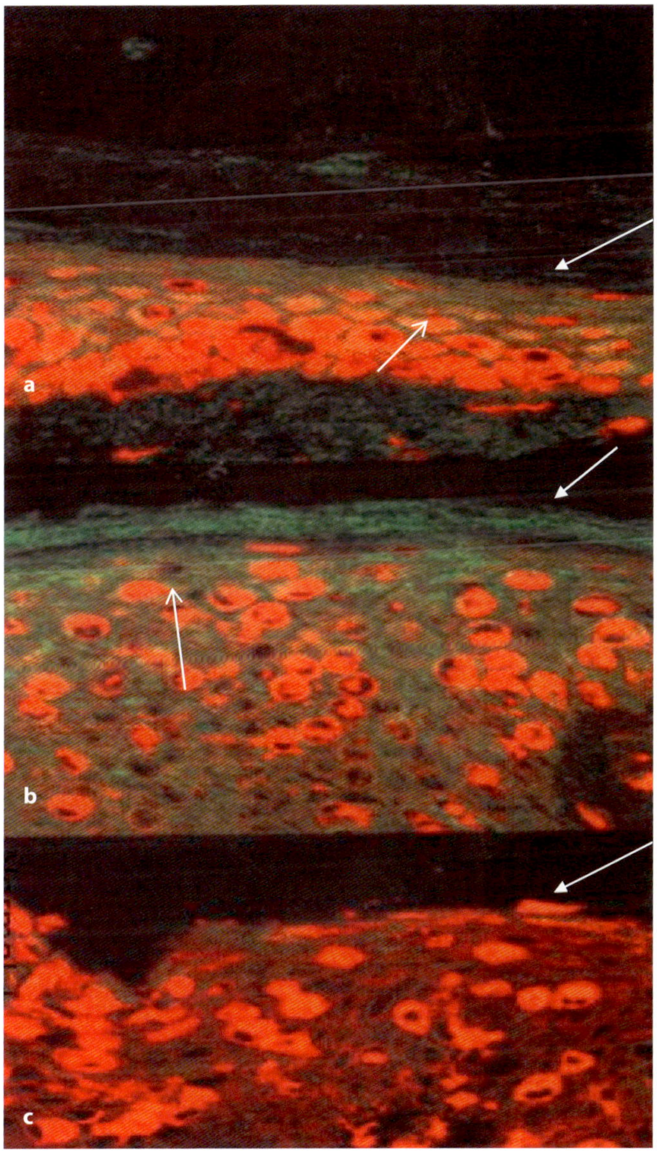

Fig. 30. Serine protease activity in normal versus RXLI skin: in situ zymography shows serine protease activity (arrows) in outer epidermis of normal, but not in RXLI frozen sections (**a**, **b**). Likewise, exogenous cholesterol sulfate inhibits serine protease activity in normal SC (**c**) (modified from Elias et al. [94]).

signs and symptoms of their systemic lipidosis, including CNS involvement, organomegaly and respiratory failure [204]. While these infants often die in the perinatal period due to progressive neurological deterioration, in surviving infants, as the collodion membrane is shed, the skin becomes near-normal, exhibiting only mild or focal scaling [98, 206]. A similar clinical phenotype is seen in a murine model homozygous for a null mutation of the β-glucocerebrosidase gene, and also in mice treated with the β-glucocerebrosidase inhibitor conduritol B epoxide, but only if enzyme activity is reduced by ≥95% [207]. Interestingly, Niemann-Pick disease, which is caused by

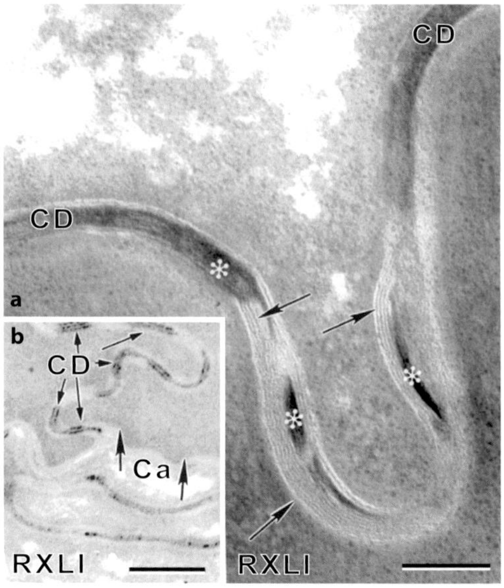

Fig. 31. Extracellular matrix abnormalities in RXLI. **a** RuO_4 postfixation, which reveals lamellar/nonlamellar (electron-dense) phase separation (asterisks). **b** Ca^{2+} leakage into the SC interstices (consistent with barrier abnormality) where it localizes to the external faces of corneodesmosomes (CD, arrows; pyroantimonate precipitation method for Ca^{2+} detection – see Appendix 1). **a** Magnification bar = 0 2 µm. **b** Magnification bar = 0 1 µm.

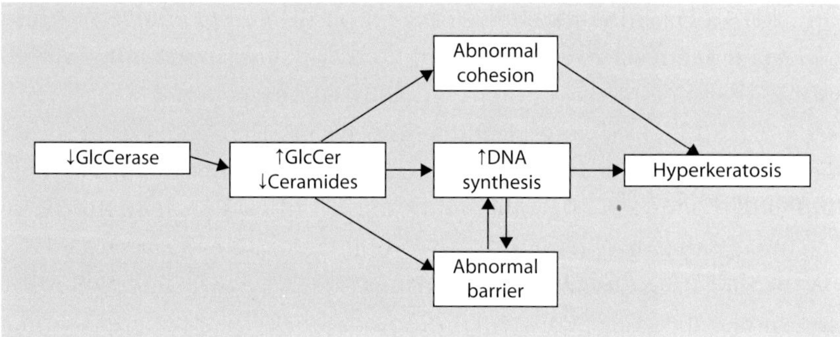

Fig. 32. Putative pathogenic mechanisms in GD. GlcCerase = Glucosylceramidase; GlcCer = glucosylceramides.

mutations in another ceramide-generating enzyme, acidic sphingomyelinase, rarely if ever manifests ichthyosiform skin changes [208, 209]. The presence of a cutaneous phenotype in GD versus the lack of a skin phenotype in Niemann-Pick disease likely reflects the generation of all known ceramides from glucosylceramides, while acidic sphingomyelinase only generates 2 ceramide fractions from corresponding sphingomyelin precursors [210].

While an ichthyosiform phenotype only occurs in the uncommon and severest type 2 or acute neuronopathic form of GD, the much more common type 1 or nonneuronopathic form of GD, which is very prevalent in the Ashkenazi Jewish population, may be asymptomatic or show signs and symptoms of lipid storage in the liver, spleen and bone marrow. Similarly, the type 3, chronic neuronopathic form, while exhibiting severer systemic symptoms, including CNS involvement, does not display an ichthyosiform phenotype. Thus, it is likely that only a severe disruption of β-glucocerebrosidase function, i.e. a null mutation, will generate a skin phenotype in GD.

Subcellular Pathogenesis

Ceramides represent 1 of the 3 key bulk lipids of the epidermal permeability barrier (in addition to FFA and cholesterol). Ceramides comprise approximately 50% of the lipids in the extracellular lamellar membranes in the SC by weight, and therefore, not surprisingly, they are absolutely required for normal barrier function [211]. Studies in type 2 GD patients, transgenic murine analogues as well as in inhibitor-based models all have shown that extreme reductions in lysosomal β-glucocerebrosidase (EC3.2.1.45) provoke a profound barrier abnormality [98, 212], but as noted above, ichthyotic signs only emerge when β- glucocerebrosidase levels are very low (<5–10% of normal) [204–206, 212].

Because topical ceramides normalize neither barrier function nor membrane ultrastructure in the face of blockade of β-glucocerebrosidase [212], the cause of the barrier abnormality in GD is complex. Both decreased ceramides, in relation to cholesterol and FFA, and accumulation of glucosylceramidase [209, 213] likely result in lamellar/nonlamellar phase separation in GD, analogous to the accumulation of another polar lipid precursor, cholesterol sulfate with reduced cholesterol, in RXLI [94] (see above). This conclusion is supported by the observation that in contrast to GD, topical ceramides normalize barrier function in severe acidic sphingomyelinase deficiency, where sphingomyelin but not glucosylceramides accumulate [208]. It is also likely that the ichthyosiform dermatosis in part reflects epidermal hyperplasia consequent to a severe permeability barrier abnormality [213], as well as a direct mitogenic activity of excess glucosylceramides [214] (fig. 32).

Diagnostic Ultrastructure

Lamellar body number, structure and secretion are normal in GD (fig. 33a, b). Instead, persistence of glucosylceramides in the SC extracellular spaces imparts an 'immature' appearance to the lamellar bilayers that is quite distinctive, and this feature alone is diagnostic of GD in an appropriate clinical setting [98, 205] (fig. 34). In addition, the excess glucosylceramides in GD appear to form an electron-dense nonlamellar phase (fig. 34c, asterisks). Nonlamellar phase separation occurs in other lipid metabolic disorders (as described in this chapter), but the extreme electron density of the nonlamellar phase is almost unique in GD (but it is also seen in RXLI – see above). The presence of normal lamellar body contents and immature lamellar structures, interspersed with electron-dense, nonlamellar material is diagnostic of GD.

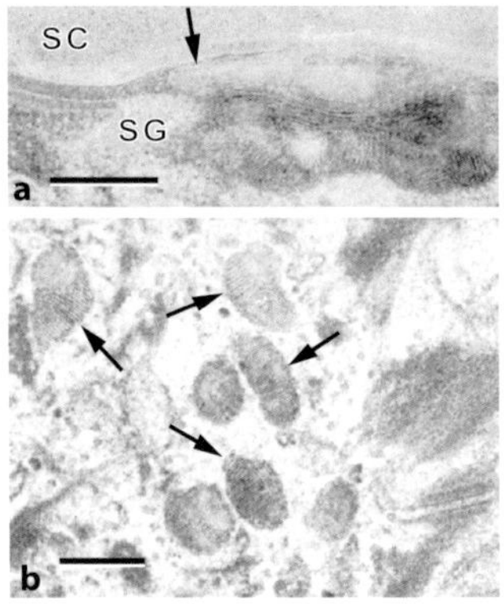

Fig. 33. Normal lamellar body density, content and secretion in GD. Magnification bars = 0.2 μm.

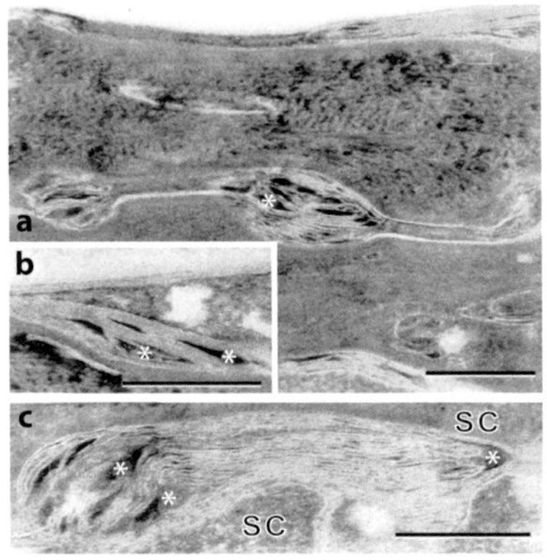

Fig. 34. Immature lamellar bilayers interspersed with electron-dense nonlamellar phase are diagnostic of GD. Asterisks indicate nonlamellar phase; arrows depict mature bilayers (rare), and normal corneocyte lipid envelope. Magnification bars = 0.2 μm. Diagnostic features: (1) incompletely processed (immature) lamellar membranes; (2) lamellar/nonlamellar phase separation with electron-dense nonlamellar phase; (3) normal lamellar body contents.

2.5. Defective Lipid Transporters

2.5.1 Ichthyosis Prematurity Syndrome

Key Clinical Features

Mothers of fetuses affected with IPS (OMIM No. 604194) experience complications early in the third trimester from polyhydramnios that culminate in premature birth at around 32 weeks. Affected infants display a thick, caseating desquamating layer that can be visualized by ultrasound in utero, resembling at birth excess vernix caseosa. Neonates with severe IPS may also experience restrictive lung disease, with asphyxia or extreme eosinophilia, which resolves over about 2 weeks. Although infants with IPS improve shortly after birth, individuals suffer from lifelong xerosis and a low-grade erythema, with minimal scaling. Atopic features, including not only dry skin, but also often severe pruritus, appear to be more prominent in females. Thus, IPS, like ichthyosis vulgaris, NLSDI and Netherton syndrome, represents another DOC in which a putative barrier abnormality can eventuate in an atopic dermatitis phenotype. In each of these entities, it is likely that either increased serine protease activation and/or sustained allergen entry across a defective SC eventually stimulates the development of a Th2 immunophenotype.

Molecular Genetics

Though IPS is most common in Scandinavia (Norway, Denmark and Finland), consistent with a founder effect [25], individual cases have been reported from North Africa, the Middle East, Germany, England and Italy. Thus, the actual prevalence of IPS may be greater than is currently estimated. All Scandinavian patients exhibit either homozygous or compound heterozygous point mutations in exon 3 on chromosome 9q34 (c.504c → a [p.C168x]) of *FATP4* or solute carrier family 27 (*SLC24A4*), also consistent with a founder effect. Mutations in this region of *FATP4* predict loss of function [25]. *FATP4* encodes a 643-amino-acid, 72-kDa peptide, with an N-terminal transmembrane binding domain [215], an endoplasmic reticulum localization signal and an AMP-binding domain (aa 243–345), consistent with its dual function as both an FFA transporter and an acylcoenzyme synthase. Thus, mutations in *FATP4* predict reduced FFA transport, with a failure of acylcoenzyme A formation.

Cellular and Molecular Pathogenesis

The epidermis expresses at least 4 members of the FATP superfamily, and in adult skin, most are regulated by permeability barrier status [216]. Yet, FATP4 is the only member of the FATP superfamily that is known to be expressed in epidermis in utero. Coincident with birth, FATP4, along with all other epidermal FATP members, rapidly upregulates [217], presumably as a compensatory response to the xeric stress imposed by the terrestrial environment. Thus, FATP4 suffices (and may be required) for the development of the epidermal barrier in utero. Since the other FATP members upregulate after birth, FATP4 may become less important, explaining the postnatal diminution of disease severity in IPS. Nevertheless, since a postnatal phenotype persists in IPS, FATP4 must still subserve an essential function for which other fatty acid transporters can only partially compensate.

Subcellular Pathogenesis

FATP4 preferentially transports very-long-chain FFA and bile acids, but its precise substrates are incompletely understood [218]. In IPS, oil red O staining and Nile red fluorescence suggest a maldistribution of neutral lipids, with accumulation in the keratinocyte cytosol, rather than secretion of lipid into the SC interstices [25]. Radiolabel studies of IPS fibroblasts show normal uptake of palmitate ($C_{16:0}$), but reduced uptake of very-long-chain FFA, such as erucic acid ($C_{22:1}$) [25]. Moreover, very-long-chain FFA fail to incorporate into glycerolipids in IPS fibroblasts. Although transport studies have not been performed with linoleate ($C_{18:2}$) or arachidonic acid ($C_{20:4}$), it is tempting to speculate that FATP4 also transports one or both of these FFA, since neither of these FFA can be synthesized by keratinocytes, which lack both the Δ^6- and Δ^9-desaturase (other tissues can synthesize arachidonic but not linoleic acid [219]). Thus, the cutaneous phenotype of IPS could reflect both the structural and proinflammatory consequences of skin-localized, essential fatty acid and/or eicosanoid deficiency [100].

Despite the diagnostic utility of intracellular lipid aggregates in IPS, they provide only a disease marker and are not of pathogenic importance, because, as in NLSDI, intracellular droplets are not bioavailable to interfere with either lamellar bilayer formation. In view of the acknowledged role of certain FATP in maintaining barrier function [216], it is highly likely, though not yet proven, that the shifting skin phenotype in adult IPS again results from pre- versus postnatal changes in permeability barrier requirements, as in HI.

Diagnostic Histology and Ultrastructure

Light microscopy reveals epidermal hyperplasia, prominent hyperkeratosis and variable inflammation with eosinophilia in the underlying dermis. Hyperkeratosis is accentuated in follicular orifices, analogous to pityriasis rubra pilaris. While these features are nondiagnostic, the presence of multiple lipid droplets in the SC on oil red O staining of frozen sections is very suggestive of IPS [25]. In contrast, lipid droplets in NLSDI are found throughout the epidermis, and in even greatest abundance in the basal layer and ducts of eccrine glands [65]. Moreover, the diagnosis of IPS can be readily made on standard electron microscopy, which reveals aggregates of curved lamellar structures in the cytosol of granular and cornified cells [220]. Hence, IPS represents a rare example of the diagnostic utility of standard light and electron microscopy without a requirement for additional RuO_4 postfixation to establish the 'diagnosis'.

The adult phenotype is associated with alterations throughout the lamellar body secretory system (fig. 35) [100]. Though the density of lamellar bodies is normal, the internal content of individual organelles often contains microvesicles (fig. 36b), as seen in NLSDI, SLS and RD. Secretion appears to be unimpaired, but vesicular material persists at the granular/cornified cell interface (fig. 36c). Although some mature lamellar bilayers form, extensive domains of lamellar/nonlamellar phase separation persist above the granular/cornified cell interface (fig. 36a), as in all the lipid metabolic disorders with ichthyosis (table 3). Although these findings suffice to both explain the persistent (putative) barrier abnormality in IPS and the adult phenotype, they are not in themselves diagnostic.

2.5.2 Harlequin Ichthyosis (Autosomal Recessive Congenital Ichthyosis)

Clinical Diagnosis

HI (OMIM No. 242500) is a rare, recessively inherited disorder that presents at birth with a thick, plate-like encasement of the entire skin surface, interrupted

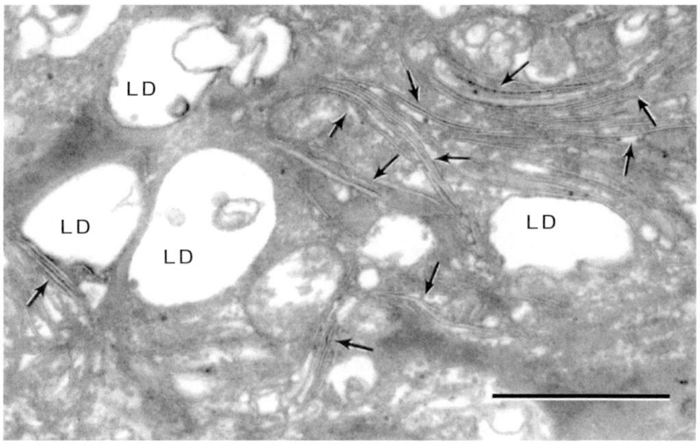

Fig. 35. The diagnostic ultrastructural features of IPS. Note lipid droplets (LD) interspersed with curved and linear arrays of lamellar material (arrows) within corneocytes in adult IPS. OsO_4 postfixation. Magnification bar = 1 μm.

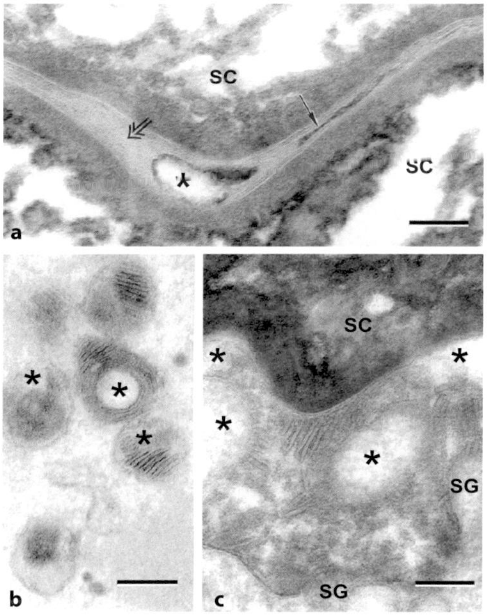

Fig. 36. Abnormalities in the lamellar body secretory system in IPS predict barrier abnormality. **b** Lamellar bodies contain microvesicles (asterisks). **c** After secretion, vesicular contents persist at the SG/SC interface (asterisks). **a** Nonlamellar/lamellar phase separation in SC interstices (asterisks; arrows indicate normal-appearing bilayers). Magnification bars = 0.1 μm.

by deep-red fissures. Severe eversion of the lips and eyelids results in a grotesque appearance. Hands and feet are encased by mitten-like scales, and the digits can appear deformed or reduced to nubbins. Yet, X-ray studies demonstrate complete bone structures under the cutaneous encasement. Infants are often born prematurely, and some are stillborn. Some HI neonates may not survive for more than a few hours or days, because constricting scales can impair respiration and/or feeding. Yet, in neonates that survive the immediate perinatal period, as the plate-like encasement is shed, the phenotype shifts to a severe ichthyosiform erythroderma [221, 222] (fig. 37).

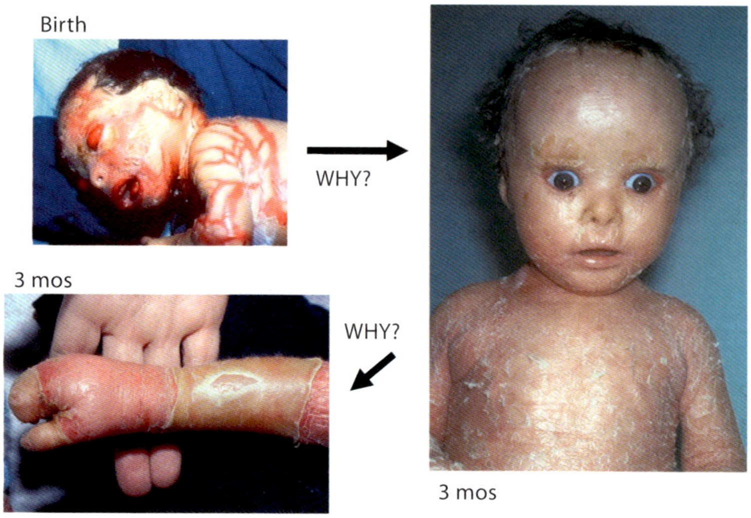

Fig. 37. HI: phenotypic shift (modified from Williams and Elias [224]). 'Phenotypic plasticity is defined as the ability of a single genotype to alter its phenotype in response to environmental conditions… important mechanism whereby populations respond rapidly to altered ecological conditions… Plasticity is ubiquitous in animal populations with traits often varying within lifetimes… depending on… conditions…' (from Nussey et al. [224]).

Biochemical Genetics

Truncation, deletion and splice junction mutations in *ABCA12* on chromosome 2q33–35 result in HI [225, 226]. ABCA12 is a member of the ABC transporter superfamily (table 4), which serves as a putative transporter for glucosylceramides from the Golgi apparatus into epidermal lamellar bodies [227]. The ABCA represent a large family of proteins that mediate transport of a variety of different lipid substrates across cell membranes. These proteins contain 2 transmembrane sequences and 2 ATP-binding domains, which undergo conformational changes that facilitate initial substrate binding, followed then by dissociation of attached lipids after transmembrane transport [228]. To date, 48 *ABC* genes have been identified, which have been further divided into 7 subfamilies, based on sequence homology and supramolecular organization of the nucleotide binding sites [225, 229–231]. The ABCA subfamily comprises 12 transporters that all mediate lipid transport (cited in Jiang et al. [232]), with the exception of 1 pseudogene (ABCA11). The ABCA are components of highly specialized lipid transporting organelles, and mutations in these transporters underlie inherited diseases affecting the cardiovascular, visual, respiratory and cutaneous organ systems (table 4).

Typically in HI, homozygous truncation or deletion mutations result in loss of function of both alleles for the gene that encodes ABCA12 [225, 226, 233], but some patients have 1 loss-of-function and 1 missense mutation [10, 225]. These mutations result in a failure to deliver newly synthesized glucosylceramides into nascent epidermal lamellar bodies (fig. 38) [225]. As a result, few if any lipids are delivered to the

Table 4. The ABCA subfamily: expression sites, function and associated diseases

Member	Expression site(s)	Putative function	Associated disorders
ABCA1	blood vessels	cholesterol, phospholipid transport	Tangier disease, familial hypoalphalipoproteinemia, early-onset atherosclerosis
ABCA2	brain, oligodendrocyte		
ABCA3	lung, alveolar type 2 cells	lamellar body lipid transport	fatal surfactant deficiency
ABCA4	eye, retinal rod cells	retinoid transport	Stargardt disease, age-related macular dystrophy, retinitis pigmentosa, cone-rod dystrophy
ABCA5	skeletal muscle	–	–
ABCA6	liver	–	–
ABCA7	spleen, hematopoietic tissue	–	–
ABCA8	ovary	–	–
ABCA9	heart	–	–
ABCA10	skeletal muscle	–	–
ABCA12	skin: epidermal keratinocytes	glucosylceramide transport into lamellar bodies	harlequin ichthyosis

SC interstices [234], resulting in a profound barrier abnormality [89]. HI keratinocytes demonstrate defective glucosylceramide transport into lamellar bodies, while conversely, transfection of the *ABCA12* gene into HI keratinocytes normalizes glucosylceramide loading [225, 235]. While the *ABCA12* mutations in HI result in loss of function, biallelic missense mutations cause a milder form of ARCI with a lamellar ichthyosis phenotype [20, 24, 225]. Since activators of 2 nuclear hormone receptors, liver X receptor and PPAR-β/δ, upregulate ABCA12 expression in normal keratinocytes [232], topical treatment with ligands of either of these receptors might benefit ARCI patients with residual ABCA12 expression.

Cellular Pathogenesis and Diagnostic Ultrastructure

Transcutaneous water loss rates remain extremely high in surviving HI patients [89], explaining in part the prominent epidermal hyperplasia and hyperkeratosis. The barrier defect in HI represents a primary disorder of the lamellar body secretory system.

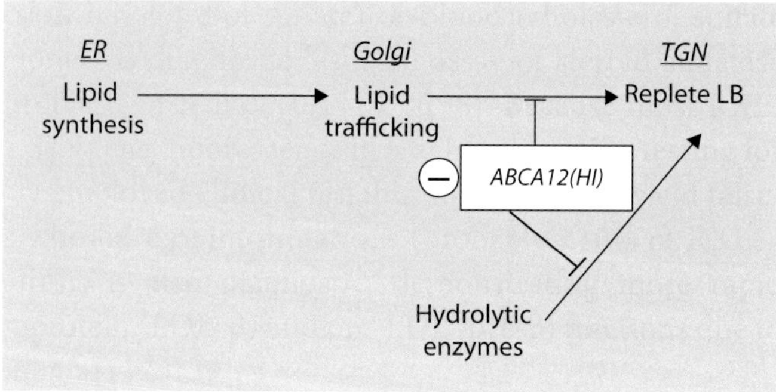

Fig. 38. Subcellular pathogenesis of HI. ER = Endoplasmic reticulum; TGN = trans-Golgi network; LB = lamellar bodies.

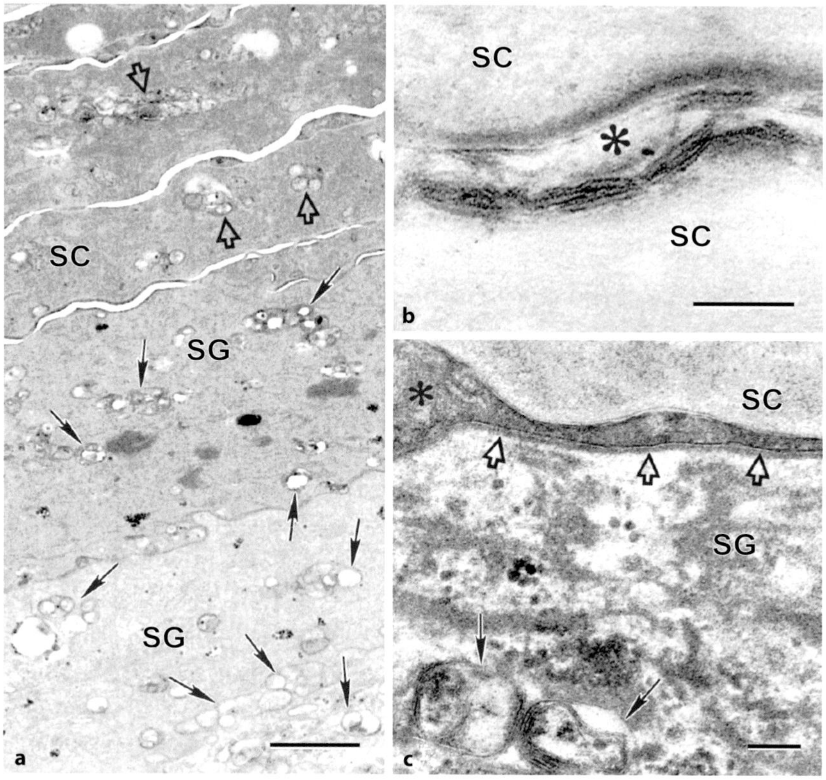

Fig. 39. Abnormal lamellar body secretory system in HI. **a** Note vesicular organelles in granular cell cytosol (arrows) and partial failure of secretion, with entombed organelles in corneocytes (open arrows). **b**, **c** Little lamellar material in extracellular spaces, which instead contain amorphous material (asterisks). **c** Although only amorphous material is apparent in SC interstices, the corneocyte lipid envelope is normal (open arrows). **a**, **c** Note sparse lamellar contents in lamellar-body-like organelles (arrows). **a** Magnification bar = 1 µm. **b**, **c** Magnification bars = 0.1 µm.

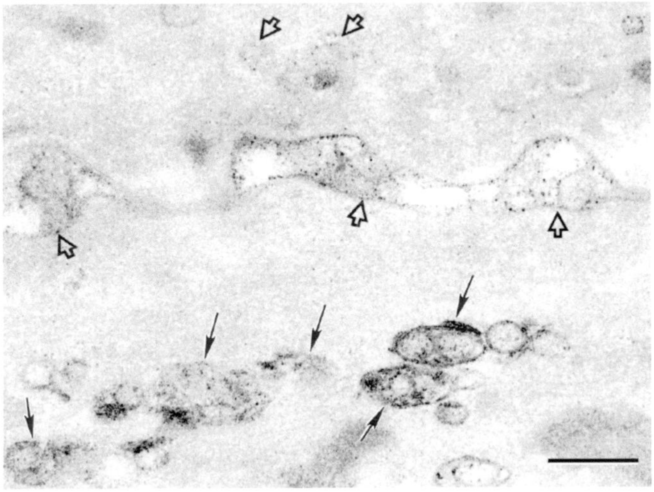

Fig. 40. Lipase ultracytochemistry in HI. Although vesicles display little or no lamellar material, they contain the hydrolases, acid lipase, a lamellar body cargo marker (arrows). Note reduced delivery of lipase to the extracellular spaces, with entombment of substantial enzyme activity in nascent corneocytes (open arrows). Magnification bar = 0.1 μm.

Specifically, lamellar bodies with replete lamellar contents are found only rarely in HI [236, 237]. Instead, the cytosol of the SG layer contains numerous vesicular structures [234], which presumably represent nascent lamellar bodies with little or no internal contents (fig. 39a, c, arrows), but it is likely that these nascent organelles undergo exocytosis, since the cornified lipid envelope, a structure thought to derive from fusion of lamellar bodies with the plasma membrane [238], is normal in HI (fig. 39b, c, open arrows) [234], and lipase cytochemistry revels low levels of secreted lamellar-body-derived hydrolytic enzymes in the extracellular spaces (fig. 40). Nevertheless, the extracellular spaces of the SC are largely devoid of lamellar membranes (fig. 39b, c) [234].

In summary, electron microscopy is diagnostic of HI. By standard electron microscopy, the SG lacks lamellar bodies with replete lamellar contents [236, 237, 239], reflecting reduced expression of the ABCA12 transporter. Yet, the cytosol of granular cells contains numerous vesicular structures that represent *forme fruste* lamellar bodies, and corneocytes display a normal corneocyte-bound lipid envelope. Reduced lamellar body contents impart a second diagnostic feature of HI, i.e. a paucity of extracellular lamellar bilayers [234, 239]. Absence of lamellar bilayers correlates with the severe barrier abnormality in HI [89]. While these observations are diagnostic of HI, it is possible that some ARCI patients with missense mutations in *ABCA12* could also display certain of these features.

A final key feature of HI is the persistence of corneodesmosomes into the outer SC, presumably due to reduced delivery of lamellar-body-derived proteases (fig. 41). HI is characterized not only by a profound barrier abnormality, but also by striking hyperkeratosis (thickening of the SC), which could represent a compensatory response to the lack of a lipid-based barrier (fig. 41). The defective lipid transporter could contribute to the desquamation abnormality, because prior cholesterol delivery

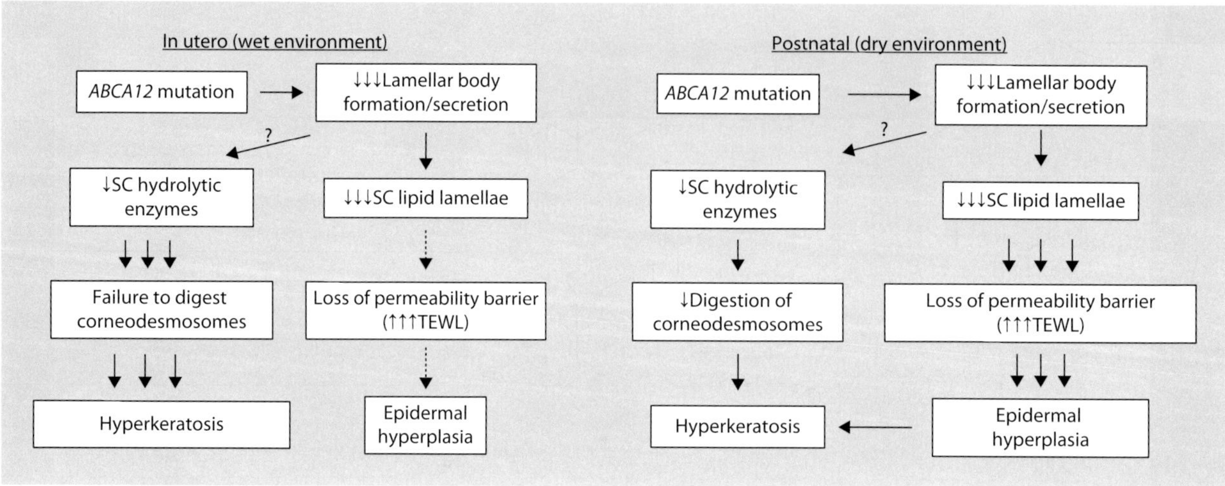

Fig. 41. 'Phenotypic shift' in HI. TEWL = Transepidermal water loss.

to lamellar bodies is required for subsequent/concurrent importation of proteins into these organelles [240]. Whether decreased glucosylceramide delivery would also impair delivery of desquamatory hydrolases, which are required for normal desquamation [241–244], to extracellular domains in HI is plausible, but unproven (fig. 38). Thus, this failure of protease delivery could result in corneodesmosome retention explaining the extreme hyperkeratosis in newborns with HI.

As in other DOC, the phenotypic shift from the neonatal to the postnatal pattern results from a homeostatic attempt to provide a competent permeability barrier (fig. 37). Because these responses are 'turned off' in the aqueous intrauterine environment, the characteristic phenotype of dense, deforming scales is present, reflecting the failure to deliver sufficient proteases to allow normal desquamation. Following birth, barrier failure drives an intense effort to compensate with pronounced epidermal hyperplasia and hyperkeratosis, with a shift to an ichthyosiform erythroderma (fig. 41). Cytochemical studies show that release of the contents of nascent lamellar bodies likely delivers sufficient proteases to ameliorate the hyperkeratosis to some extent (fig. 40); lamellar body secretion is stimulated by barrier repair signals. This pathogenic sequence is supported by the observation that the phenotype reverts to the in utero pattern, when postnatal skin is occluded (i.e. fully hydrated) under an orthopedic cast (fig. 37).

2.5.3 CEDNIK, MEDNIK and ARC Syndromes

Clinical Features and Biochemical Genetics

CEDNIK Syndrome (OMIM No. 609528). This is a recessively inherited disorder with ichthyosis, characterized by failure to thrive and developmental retardation, hence the acronym cerebral dysgenesis, neuropathy, ichthyosis and keratoderma (CEDNIK) syndrome. This noncongenital neurocutaneous syndrome, with microcephaly, mental retardation, sensorineural deafness, generalized ichthyosis and palmar-plantar keratoderma, was recently ascribed to mutations in the *SNAP29* gene, encoding for the soluble N-ethylmaleimide-sensitive factor attachment protein receptor (SNARE) 29 protein, which is involved in intracellular vesicle fusion [245]. The key cutaneous features are palmar-plantar keratoderma and generalized scaling, which reportedly appear between 5 and 11 months [245].

MEDNIK Syndrome (OMIM No. 609313). MEDNIK syndrome, with mental retardation, enteropathy (severe diarrhea), deafness, peripheral neuropathy, ichthyosis and keratoderma, is a recessively inherited disorder, described to date solely in 3 French-Canadian families. The skin presents as an atypical erythrokeratoderma-variabilis-like dermatosis with palmar-plantar keratoderma [246]. The disease is recessively inherited due to a mutation in the *AP1S1* gene on chromosome 7q22, which encodes a subunit of an AP-1 that shuttles proteins between the trans-Golgi network, the endosomal pathway and the plasma membrane [247]. The overall clinical picture resembles CEDNIK syndrome, and the pathogenesis of the cutaneous phenotype is likely similar (see below).

ARC Syndrome (OMIM No. 208085). Arthogryposis, renal dysfunction and cholestasis (ARC) syndrome is a rare, lethal, autosomal recessive, multisystem disorder. Loss-of-function mutations in the *VPS33B* gene underlie ARC syndrome [248]. *VPS33B* encodes the vacuolar protein-sorting protein Vps33, which regulates vesicle-to-target SNARE complex formation during exocytosis [247, 249]. Thus, Vps33 deficiency, like SNARE29 and AP-1 deficiency, presumably impairs lamellar body secretion.

Most cases include multiple congenital abnormalities of variable severity, including a severe lamellar-type ichthyosis [250]. At birth, patients display normal pink skin, a small head circumference, facial dysmorphism, low-set ears and multiple limb contractures or arthrogryposis, primarily of the elbows and knees as a result of decreased fetal movements, as well as club or 'rocker-bottom' feet [250–253]. Clinically and radiographically, patients display narrow ribs, osteopenia and rickets. Widening of the kidney collecting system, with severe renal tubular dysfunction, aminoaciduria, glycosuria, renal tubular acidosis and nephrogenic diabetes insipidus and/or renal calcification also occur [250]. While severe renal failure could explain failure to thrive in these patients, the severe ichthyosiform dermatitis is also likely to be contributory. By 6 weeks, patients display widespread LI, involving the trunk, scalp and extremities, with sparing of the face and palmoplantar surfaces. In addition, cholestatic jaundice occurs, with hyperbilirubinemia and markedly elevated alkaline phosphatase levels. The clinical course of ARC syndrome is dominated by recurrent infections, diarrhea, dehydration, severe failure to thrive and metabolic acidosis. Despite treatment with medium-chain triglycerides, fat-soluble vitamins, ursodecholic acid and/or sodium bicarbonate, patients fail to gain weight or achieve any developmental milestones, and succumb before 1 year of age [249, 251].

Ultrastructural Pathology

CEDNIK Syndrome. A large body of evidence supports the concept that lamellar bodies originate from the trans-Golgi complex [254]. Accordingly, a number of studies have shown that SNAP29, in contrast to other SNAP proteins [255, 256], locates predominantly to intracellular membrane structures [257–259], suggesting a specific role for SNAP29 in mediating trafficking out of the trans-Golgi network [260]. The most striking ultrastructural abnormality in CEDNIK epidermis is the presence of abundant empty or partially empty vesicles (presumed *forme fruste* lamellar bodies) in the spinous and granular layers by standard electron microscopy [245]. Vesicles of various sizes and contents are also retained in corneocytes, suggesting a failure of lamellar body secretion, with entombment of unsecreted lamellar body contents.

ARC and MEDNIK Syndromes. VPS33B is thought to regulate SNARE-mediated vesicle secretion [247], including neuromediator secretion [261]. While lamellar body maturation is normal in ARC syndrome by standard electron microscopy, lamellar body secretion is abnormal [249]. Moreover, while lamellar body internal structure is normal, numerous lamellar bodies are retained within cornified cells, as in CEDNIK syndrome. Thus, *VPS33B* mutations could cause a permeability barrier abnormality by impairing lamellar body secretion. However, the defect could be limited to a subset of lamellar bodies in the epidermis, explaining the selective enrichment of glucosylceramide, kallikrein 5 and kallikrein 7 in retained vesicular structures that resemble lamellar bodies (see below).

Although there are no ultrastructural studies to date, the general role of AP-1 in vesicular secretion would predict that a lamellar body secretory defect likely occurs in MEDNIK syndrome as well. Thus, ARC, CEDNIK and MEDNIK syndromes appear to result from abnormal function of proteins involved in vesicle secretion [247, 248, 257], which in epidermis would lead to impaired lamellar body exocytosis. Together, these observations suggest that VPS33B likely regulates lamellar body exocytosis, while AP1S1 and SNAP29 are involved in vesicle transport within or out of the trans-Golgi network in preparation for secretion [249].

2.6. References

1 Swanbeck G: The ichthyosis. Acta Derm Venereol Suppl (Stockh) 1981;95:88–90.

2 Williams ML, Elias PM: Heterogeneity in autosomal recessive ichthyosis: clinical and biochemical differentiation of lamellar ichthyosis and nonbullous congenital ichthyosiform erythroderma. Arch Dermatol 1985;121:477–488.

3 Arnold ML, Anton-Lamprecht I, Melz-Rothfuss B, Hartschuh W: Ichthyosis congenita type III: clinical and ultrastructural characteristics and distinction within the heterogeneous ichthyosis congenita group. Arch Dermatol Res 1988;280:268–278.

4 Ghadially R, Williams ML, Hou SY, Elias PM: Membrane structural abnormalities in the stratum corneum of the autosomal recessive ichthyoses. J Invest Dermatol 1992;99:755–763.

5 Eckl KM, de Juanes S, Kurtenbach J, et al: Molecular analysis of 250 patients with autosomal recessive congenital ichthyosis: evidence for mutation hotspots in ALOXE3 and allelic heterogeneity in ALOX12B. J Invest Dermatol 2009;129:1421–1428.

6 Russell LJ, Di Giovanna JJ, Rogers GR, et al: Mutations in the gene for transglutaminase 1 in autosomal recessive lamellar ichthyosis. Nat Genet 1995;9:279–283.
7 Huber M, Rettler I, Bernasconi K, et al: Mutations of keratinocyte transglutaminase in lamellar ichthyosis. Science 1995;267:525–528.
8 Hennies HC, Kuster W, Wiebe V, Krebsova A, Reis A: Genotype/phenotype correlation in autosomal recessive lamellar ichthyosis. Am J Hum Genet 1998;62:1052–1061.
9 Jobard F, Lefevre C, Karaduman A, et al: Lipoxygenase-3 (ALOXE3) and 12R-lipoxygenase (ALOX12B) are mutated in non-bullous congenital ichthyosiform erythroderma (NCIE) linked to chromosome 17p13.1. Hum Mol Genet 2002;11:107–113.
10 Akiyama M, Sawamura D, Shimizu H: The clinical spectrum of nonbullous congenital ichthyosiform erythroderma and lamellar ichthyosis. Clin Exp Dermatol 2003;28:235–240.
11 Vahlquist A, Ganemo A, Pigg M, Virtanen M, Westermark P: The clinical spectrum of congenital ichthyosis in Sweden: a review of 127 cases. Acta Derm Venereol Suppl (Stockh) 2003;83:34–47.
12 Eckl KM, Krieg P, Kuster W, et al: Mutation spectrum and functional analysis of epidermis-type lipoxygenases in patients with autosomal recessive congenital ichthyosis. Hum Mutat 2005;26:351–361.
13 Fischer J, Faure A, Bouadjar B, et al: Two new loci for autosomal recessive ichthyosis on chromosomes 3p21 and 19p12–q12 and evidence for further genetic heterogeneity. Am J Hum Genet 2000;66: 904–913.
14 Richard G: Molecular genetics of the ichthyoses. Am J Med Genet C Semin Med Genet 2004;131C:32–44.
15 Anton-Lamprecht I: Ultrastructural identification of basic abnormalities as clues to genetic disorders of the epidermis. J Invest Dermatol 1994;103:6S–12S.
16 Williams ML: Ichthyosis: mechanisms of disease. Pediatr Dermatol 1992;9:365–368.
17 Williams ML: Epidermal lipids and scaling diseases of the skin. Semin Dermatol 1992;11:169–175.
18 Fischer J: Autosomal recessive congenital ichthyosis. J Invest Dermatol 2009;129:1319–1321.
19 Elias PM, Williams ML, Holleran WM, Jiang YJ, Schmuth M: Pathogenesis of permeability barrier abnormalities in the ichthyoses: inherited disorders of lipid metabolism. J Lipid Res 2008;49:697–714.
20 Lefevre C, Audebert S, Jobard F, et al: Mutations in the transporter ABCA12 are associated with lamellar ichthyosis type 2. Hum Mol Genet 2003;12:2369–2378.
21 Vahlquist A, Bygum A, Ganemo A, et al: Genotypic and clinical spectrum of self-improving collodion ichthyosis: *ALOX12B, ALOXE3,* and *TGM1* mutations in Scandinavian patients. J Invest Dermatol 2010;130:438–443.
22 Farasat S, Wei MH, Herman M, et al: Novel transglutaminase-1 mutations and genotype-phenotype investigations of 104 patients with autosomal recessive congenital ichthyosis in the USA. J Med Genet 2009;46:103–111.
23 Harting M, Brunetti-Pierri N, Chan CS, et al: Self-healing collodion membrane and mild nonbullous congenital ichthyosiform erythroderma due to 2 novel mutations in the *ALOX12B* gene. Arch Dermatol 2008;144:351–356.
24 Hohl D, Williams ML: Ichthyoses and related mendelian disorders of cornification (MEDOC); in Irvine A, Hoger P, Yan A (eds): Textbook of Pediatric Dermatology. In press.
25 Klar J, Schweiger M, Zimmerman R, et al: Mutations in the fatty acid transport protein 4 gene cause the ichthyosis prematurity syndrome. Am J Hum Genet 2009;85:248–253.
26 Sakai K, Akiyama M, Yanagi T, et al: *ABCA12* is a major causative gene for non-bullous congenital ichthyosiform erythroderma. J Invest Dermatol 2009;129:2306–2309.
27 Hallopeau H, Watelet R: Sur une forme atténuée de la maladie dite ichtyose fœtale. Ann Dermatol Syphilol 1884;3:149–152.
28 Van Gysel D, Lijnen RL, Moekti SS, de Laat PC, Oranje AP: Collodion baby: a follow-up study of 17 cases. J Eur Acad Dermatol Venereol 2002;16:472–475.
29 Lawlor F: Progress of a harlequin fetus to non-bullous ichthyosiform erythroderma. Pediatrics 1988;82:870–873.
30 Lefevre C, Bouadjar B, Karaduman A, et al: Mutations in ichthyin a new gene on chromosome 5q33 in a new form of autosomal recessive congenital ichthyosis. Hum Mol Genet 2004;13:2473–2482.
31 Lesueur F, Bouadjar B, Lefevre C, et al: Novel mutations in *ALOX12B* in patients with autosomal recessive congenital ichthyosis and evidence for genetic heterogeneity on chromosome 17p13. J Invest Dermatol 2007;127:829–834.
32 Dahlqvist J, Klar J, Hausser I, et al: Congenital ichthyosis: mutations in ichthyin are associated with specific structural abnormalities in the granular layer of epidermis. J Med Genet 2007;44:615–620.
33 Zeeuwen PL, Cheng T, Schalkwijk J: The biology of cystatin M/E and its cognate target proteases. J Invest Dermatol 2009;129:1327–1338.
34 Oji V, Zeeuwen P, Schalkwijk J, Traupe H: Evaluation of cystatin M/E: a candidate for cornification disorders. Arch Dermatol Res 2005;296:408.

35 Anton R, Vila L: Stereoselective biosynthesis of hepoxilin B3 in human epidermis. J Invest Dermatol 2000;114:554–559.
36 Anton R, Camacho M, Puig L, Vila L: Hepoxilin B3 and its enzymatically formed derivative trioxilin B3 are incorporated into phospholipids in psoriatic lesions. J Invest Dermatol 2002;118:139–146.
37 Krieg P, Marks F, Furstenberger G: A gene cluster encoding human epidermis-type lipoxygenases at chromosome 17p13.1: cloning, physical mapping, and expression. Genomics 2001;73:323–330.
38 Yu Z, Schneider C, Boeglin WE, Marnett LJ, Brash AR: The lipoxygenase gene *ALOXE3* implicated in skin differentiation encodes a hydroperoxide isomerase. Proc Natl Acad Sci USA 2003;100:9162–9167.
39 Yu Z, Schneider C, Boeglin WE, Brash AR: Mutations associated with a congenital form of ichthyosis (NCIE) inactivate the epidermal lipoxygenases 12R-LOX and eLOX3. Biochim Biophys Acta 2005; 16863:238–247.
40 Epp N, Furstenberger G, Muller K, et al: 12R-Lipoxygenase deficiency disrupts epidermal barrier function. J Cell Biol 2007;177:173–182.
41 Moran JL, Qiu H, Turbe-Doan A, et al: A mouse mutation in the 12R-lipoxygenase, Alox12b, disrupts formation of the epidermal permeability barrier. J Invest Dermatol 2007;127:1893–1897.
42 Schmuth M, Gruber R, Elias PM, Williams M: Ichthyosis update: towards a function-driven model of pathogenesis of the disorders of cornification and the role of corneocyte proteins in these disorders. Adv Dermatol 2007;23:231–256.
43 Lefevre C, Bouadjar B, Ferrand V, et al: Mutations in a new cytochrome P450 gene in lamellar ichthyosis type 3. Hum Mol Genet 2006;15:767–776.
44 Brash AR, Yu Z, Boeglin WE, Schneider C: The hepoxilin connection in the epidermis. FEBS J 2007; 274:3494–3502.
45 Williams ML, Coleman RA, Placezk D, Grunfeld C: Neutral lipid storage disease: a possible functional defect in phospholipid-linked triacylglycerol metabolism. Biochim Biophys Acta 1991;1096:162–169.
46 Schweiger M, Lass A, Zimmermann R, Eichmann TO, Zechner R: Neutral lipid storage disease: genetic disorders caused by mutations in adipose triglyceride lipase/PNPLA2 or CGI-58/ABHD5. Am J Physiol Endocrinol Metab 2009;297:E289–E296.
47 Elias PM, Brown BE: The mammalian cutaneous permeability barrier: defective barrier function is essential fatty acid deficiency correlates with abnormal intercellular lipid deposition. Lab Invest 1978; 39:574–583.
48 Elias PM, Brown BE, Ziboh VA: The permeability barrier in essential fatty acid deficiency: evidence for a direct role for linoleic acid in barrier function. J Invest Dermatol 1980;74:230–233.
49 Nugteren DH, Christ-Hazelhof E, van der Beek A, Houtsmuller UM: Metabolism of linoleic acid and other essential fatty acids in the epidermis of the rat. Biochim Biophys Acta 1985;834:429–436.
50 Hou SY, Mitra AK, White SH, Menon GK, Ghadially R, Elias PM: Membrane structures in normal and essential fatty acid-deficient stratum corneum: characterization by ruthenium tetroxide staining and X-ray diffraction. J Invest Dermatol 1991;96: 215–223.
51 Yu Z, Schneider C, Boeglin WE, Brash AR: Epidermal lipoxygenase products of the hepoxilin pathway selectively activate the nuclear receptor PPARalpha. Lipids 2007;42:491–497.
52 Rivier M, Safonova I, Lebrun P, Griffiths CE, Ailhaud G, Michel S: Differential expression of peroxisome proliferator-activated receptor subtypes during the differentiation of human keratinocytes. J Invest Dermatol 1998;111:1116–1121.
53 Hanley K, Jiang Y, He SS, et al: Keratinocyte differentiation is stimulated by activators of the nuclear hormone receptor PPARalpha. J Invest Dermatol 1998;110:368–375.
54 Sheu MY, Fowler AJ, Kao J, et al: Topical peroxisome proliferator activated receptor-alpha activators reduce inflammation in irritant and allergic contact dermatitis models. J Invest Dermatol 2002; 118:94–101.
55 Schmuth M, Schoonjans K, Yu QC, et al: Role of peroxisome proliferator-activated receptor alpha in epidermal development in utero. J Invest Dermatol 2002;119:1298–1303.
56 Dubrac S, Stoitzner P, Pirkebner D, et al: Peroxisome proliferator-activated receptor-alpha activation inhibits Langerhans cell function. J Immunol 2007;178: 4362–4372.
57 Cowart LA, Wei S, Hsu MH, et al: The CYP4A isoforms hydroxylate epoxyeicosatrienoic acids to form high affinity peroxisome proliferator-activated receptor ligands. J Biol Chem 2002;277:35105–35112.
58 Reynaud D, Demin PM, Sutherland M, Nigam S, Pace-Asciak CR: Hepoxilin signaling in intact human neutrophils: biphasic elevation of intracellular calcium by unesterified hepoxilin A3. FEBS Lett 1999;446:236–238.
59 Lavrijsen AP, Bouwstra JA, Gooris GS, Weerheim A, Bodde HE, Ponec M: Reduced skin barrier function parallels abnormal stratum corneum lipid organization in patients with lamellar ichthyosis. J Invest Dermatol 1995;105:619–624.

60 Elias PM, Schmuth M, Uchida Y, et al: Basis for the permeability barrier abnormality in lamellar ichthyosis. Exp Dermatol 2002;11:248–256.
61 De Juanes S, Epp N, Latzko S, et al: Development of an ichthyosiform phenotype in Alox12b-deficient mouse skin transplants. J Invest Dermatol 2009;129: 1429–1436.
62 Ganemo A, Pigg M, Virtanen M, et al: Autosomal recessive congenital ichthyosis in Sweden and Estonia: clinical, genetic and ultrastructural findings in eighty-three patients. Acta Derm Venereol 2003;83:24–30.
63 Bouwstra JA, Ponec M: The skin barrier in healthy and diseased state. Biochim Biophys Acta 2006; 1758:2080–2095.
64 4Natsuga K, Akiyama M, Kato N, et al: Novel *ABCA12* mutations identified in two cases of non-bullous congenital ichthyosiform erythroderma associated with multiple skin malignant neoplasia. J Invest Dermatol 2007;127:2669–2673.
65 Elias PM, Williams ML: Neutral lipid storage disease with ichthyosis: defective lamellar body contents and intracellular dispersion. Arch Dermatol 1985;121:1000–1008.
66 Demerjian M, Crumrine DA, Milstone LM, Williams ML, Elias PM: Barrier dysfunction and pathogenesis of neutral lipid storage disease with ichthyosis (Chanarin-Dorfman syndrome). J Invest Dermatol 2006;126:2032–2038.
67 Williams ML, Koch TK, McDonnell JJ, et al: Ichthyosis and neutral-lipid storage disease. Am J Med Genet 1985;20:711–726.
68 Pujol RM, Gilaberte M, Toll A, et al: Erythrokeratoderma variabilis-like ichthyosis in Chanarin-Dorfman syndrome. Br J Dermatol 2005;153: 838–841.
69 Solomon C, Bernier L, Germain L, Dufour R, Davignon J: Severe oily ichthyosis in monozygotic twins mimicking Chanarin-Dorfman syndrome but not associated with a mutation of the CGI58 gene. Arch Dermatol 2006;142:402–403.
70 Ujihara M, Nakajima K, Yamamoto M, et al: Epidermal triglyceride levels are correlated with severity of ichthyosis in Dorfman-Chanarin syndrome. J Dermatol Sci 20010;57:102–107.
71 Lefevre C, Jobard F, Caux F, et al: Mutations in CGI-58, the gene encoding a new protein of the esterase/lipase/thioesterase subfamily, in Chanarin-Dorfman syndrome. Am J Hum Genet 2001;69:1002–1012.
72 Akiyama M, Sawamura D, Nomura Y, Sugawara M, Shimizu H: Truncation of CGI-58 protein causes malformation of lamellar granules resulting in ichthyosis in Dorfman-Chanarin syndrome. J Invest Dermatol 2003;121:1029–1034.
73 Ben Selma Z, Yilmaz S, Schischmanoff PO, et al: A novel S115G mutation of CGI-58 in a Turkish patient with Dorfman-Chanarin syndrome. J Invest Dermatol 2007;127:2273–2276.
74 Fischer J, Lefevre C, Morava E, et al: The gene encoding adipose triglyceride lipase (PNPLA2) is mutated in neutral lipid storage disease with myopathy. Nat Genet 2007;39:28–30.
75 Lass A, Zimmermann R, Haemmerle G, et al: Adipose triglyceride lipase-mediated lipolysis of cellular fat stores is activated by CGI-58 and defective in Chanarin-Dorfman syndrome. Cell Metab 2006;3: 309–319.
76 Radner FP, Streith IE, Schoiswohl G, et al: Growth retardation, impaired triacylglycerol catabolism, hepatic steatosis, and lethal skin barrier defect in mice lacking comparative gene identification-58 (CGI-58). J Biol Chem 20010;285:7300–7311.
77 Igal RA, Coleman RA: Acylglycerol recycling from triacylglycerol to phospholipid, not lipase activity, is defective in neutral lipid storage disease fibroblasts. J Biol Chem 1996;271:16644–16651.
78 Igal RA, Coleman RA: Neutral lipid storage disease: a genetic disorder with abnormalities in the regulation of phospholipid metabolism. J Lipid Res 1998; 39:31–43.
79 Man MQ, Feingold KR, Jain M, Elias PM: Extracellular processing of phospholipids is required for permeability barrier homeostasis. J Lipid Res 1995; 36:1925–1935.
80 Fluhr JW, Elias PM: Stratum corneum pH: formation and function of the 'acid mantle'. Exog Dermatol 2002;1:163–175.
81 Elias PM, Steinhoff M: 'Outside-to-inside' (and now back to 'outside') pathogenic mechanisms in atopic dermatitis. J Invest Dermatol 2008;128:1067–1070.
82 Zaynoun ST, Aftimos BG, Tenekjian KK, Bahuth N, Kurban AK: Extensive pityriasis alba: a histological histochemical and ultrastructural study. Br J Dermatol 1983;108:83–90.
83 Johnson BL, Kramer EM, Lavker RM: The keratotic tumors of Cowden's disease: an electronmicroscopic study. J Cutan Pathol 1987;14:291–298.
84 Kanerva L: Electron microscopy of the effects of dithranol on healthy and on psoriatic skin. Am J Dermatopathol 1990;12:51–62.
85 el-Shoura SM, Tallab TM: Richner-Hanhart's syndrome: new ultrastructural observations on skin lesions of two cases. Ultrastruct Pathol 1997;21:51–56.
86 Monteiro-Riviere NA, Inman AO, Riviere JE: Skin toxicity of jet fuels: ultrastructural studies and the effects of substance P. Toxicol Appl Pharmacol 2004;195:339–347.

87 Elias PM, Menon GK: Structural and lipid biochemical correlates of the epidermal permeability barrier. Adv Lipid Res 1991;24:1–26.
88 Yamaguchi T, Omatsu N, Matsushita S, Osumi T: CGI-58 interacts with perilipin and is localized to lipid droplets: possible involvement of CGI-58 mislocalization in Chanarin-Dorfman syndrome. J Biol Chem 2004;279:30490–30497.
89 Moskowitz DG, Fowler AJ, Heyman MB, et al: Pathophysiologic basis for growth failure in children with ichthyosis: an evaluation of cutaneous ultrastructure, epidermal permeability barrier function, and energy expenditure. J Pediatr 2004;145:82–92.
90 Uchida Y, Cho YH, Moradian S, et al: Neutral lipid storage leads to acylceramide deficiency, likely contributing to the pathogenesis of Dorfman-Chanarin syndrome. SID 2010 Annu Meet, Atlanta, 2010.
91 Bangham, AD: Lipid bilayers and biomembranes. Annu Rev Biochem 1972;41:753–776.
92 Rehfeld SJ, Williams ML, Elias PM: Interactions of cholesterol and cholesterol sulfate with free fatty acids: possible relevance for the pathogenesis of recessive X-linked ichthyosis. Arch Dermatol Res 1986;278:259–263.
93 Rehfeld SJ, Plachy WZ, Williams ML, Elias PM: Calorimetric and electron spin resonance examination of lipid phase transitions in human stratum corneum: molecular basis for normal cohesion and abnormal desquamation in recessive X-linked ichthyosis. J Invest Dermatol 1988;91:499–505.
94 Elias PM, Crumrine D, Rassner U, et al: Basis for abnormal desquamation and permeability barrier dysfunction in RXLI. J Invest Dermatol 2004;122: 314–319.
95 Van den Brink DM, Wanders RJ: Phytanic acid: production from phytol, its breakdown and role in human disease. Cell Mol Life Sci 2006;63:1752–1765.
96 Shibaki A, Akiyama M, Shimizu H: Novel *ALDH3A2* heterozygous mutations are associated with defective lamellar granule formation in a Japanese family of Sjögren-Larsson syndrome. J Invest Dermatol 2004;123:1197–1199.
97 Rizzo WB: Sjögren-Larsson syndrome: molecular genetics and biochemical pathogenesis of fatty aldehyde dehydrogenase deficiency. Mol Genet Metab 2007;90:1–9.
98 Holleran WM, Ziegler SG, Goker-Alpan O, et al: Skin abnormalities as an early predictor of neurologic outcome in Gaucher disease. Clin Genet 2006; 69:355–357.
99 Emami S, Hanley KP, Esterly NB, Daniallinia N, Williams ML: X-linked dominant ichthyosis with peroxisomal deficiency: an ultrastructural and ultracytochemical study of the Conradi-Hünermann syndrome and its murine homologue, the bare patches mouse. Arch Dermatol 1994;130:325–336.
100 Khnykin D, Crumrine D, Uchida Y, Johansen F, Jahnsen F, Elias P: Epidermal barrier abnormalities and pathogenesis of ichthyosis prematurity syndrome. SID 2010 Annu Meet, Atlanta, 2010.
101 Willemsen MA, Ijlst L, Steijlen PM, et al: Clinical, biochemical and molecular genetic characteristics of 19 patients with the Sjögren-Larsson syndrome. Brain 2001;124:1426–1437.
102 Jagell S, Liden S: Ichthyosis in the Sjögren-Larsson syndrome. Clin Genet 1982;21:243–252.
103 Paige DG, Morse-Fisher N, Harper JI: Quantification of stratum corneum ceramides and lipid envelope ceramides in the hereditary ichthyoses. Br J Dermatol 1994;131:23–27.
104 Wedi B, Kapp A: Pathophysiological role of leukotrienes in dermatological diseases: potential therapeutic implications. Biodrugs 2001;15:729–743.
105 Rizzo WB, Craft DA: Sjögren-Larsson syndrome: accumulation of free fatty alcohols in cultured fibroblasts and plasma. J Lipid Res 2000;41:1077–1081.
106 Rizzo WB: Sjögren-Larsson syndrome: explaining the skin-brain connection. Neurology 1999;52:1307–1308.
107 Gordon N: Sjögren-Larsson syndrome. Dev Med Child Neurol 2007;49:152–154.
108 Rizzo WB, S'Aulis D, Jennings MA, Crumrine DA, Williams ML, Elias PM: Ichthyosis in Sjögren-Larsson syndrome reflects defective barrier function due to abnormal lamellar body structure and secretion. Arch Dermatol Res 2010, E-pub ahead of print.
109 Jansen GA, Ferdinandusse S, Hogenhout EM, Verhoeven NM, Jakobs C, Wanders RJ: Phytanoyl-CoA hydroxylase deficiency: enzymological and molecular basis of classical Refsum disease. Adv Exp Med Biol 1999;466:371–376.
110 Blanchet-Bardon C, Anton-Lamprecht I, Puissant A, Schnyder U: Ultrastructural features of ichthyotic skin in Refsum's syndrome; in Marks R, Dykes P (eds): The Ichthyoses. New York, SP Medical & Scientific Books, 1978, pp 65–69.
111 Van den Brink DM, Brites P, Haasjes J, et al: Identification of *PEX7* as the second gene involved in Refsum disease. Am J Hum Genet 2003;72:471–477.
112 Pahan K, Khan M, Singh I: Phytanic acid oxidation: normal activation and transport yet defective alpha-hydroxylation of phytanic acid in peroxisomes from Refsum disease and rhizomelic chondrodysplasia punctata. J Lipid Res 1996;37:1137–1143.

113 Emami S, Rizzo WB, Hanley KP, Taylor JM, Goldyne ME, Williams ML: Peroxisomal abnormality in fibroblasts from involved skin of CHILD syndrome: case study and review of peroxisomal disorders in relation to skin disease. Arch Dermatol 1992;128: 1213–1222.
114 Verhoeven NM, Jakobs C, Carney G, Somers MP, Wanders RJ, Rizzo WB: Involvement of microsomal fatty aldehyde dehydrogenase in the alpha-oxidation of phytanic acid. FEBS Lett 1998;429:225–228.
115 Happle R: Lyonization and the lines of Blaschko. Hum Genet 1985;70:200–206.
116 Happle R: X-linked dominant chondrodysplasia punctata: review of literature and report of a case. Hum Genet 1979;53:65–73.
117 Ikegawa S, Ohashi H, Ogata T, et al: Novel and recurrent EBP mutations in X-linked dominant chondrodysplasia punctata. Am J Med Genet 2000; 94:300–305.
118 Steijlen PM, van Geel M, Vreeburg M, et al: Novel EBP gene mutations in Conradi-Hünermann-Happle syndrome. Br J Dermatol 2007;157:1225–1229.
119 Feldmeyer L, Mevorah B, Grzeschik KH, Huber M, Hohl D: Clinical variation in X-linked dominant chondrodysplasia punctata (X-linked dominant ichthyosis). Br J Dermatol 2006;154:766–769.
120 Herman GE, Kelley RI, Pureza V, et al: Characterization of mutations in 22 females with X-linked dominant chondrodysplasia punctata (Happle syndrome). Genet Med 2002;4:434–438.
121 Grange DK, Kratz LE, Braverman NE, Kelley RI: CHILD syndrome caused by deficiency of 3beta-hydroxysteroid-delta8, delta7-isomerase. Am J Med Genet 2000;90:328–335.
122 Konig A, Happle R, Bornholdt D, Engel H, Grzeschik KH: Mutations in the *NSDHL* gene, encoding a 3beta-hydroxysteroid dehydrogenase, cause CHILD syndrome. Am J Med Genet 2000;90:339–346.
123 Happle R: X-chromosome inactivation: role in skin disease expression. Acta Paediatr Suppl 2006;95:16–23.
124 Derry JM, Gormally E, Means GD, et al: Mutations in a delta 8-delta 7 sterol isomerase in the tattered mouse and X-linked dominant chondrodysplasia punctata. Nat Genet 1999;22:286–290.
125 Braverman N, Lin P, Moebius FF, et al: Mutations in the gene encoding 3 beta-hydroxysteroid-delta 8, delta 7-isomerase cause X-linked dominant Conradi-Hünermann syndrome. Nat Genet 1999;22:291–294.
126 Kelley RI, Herman GE: Inborn errors of sterol biosynthesis. Annu Rev Genomics Hum Genet 2001; 2:299–341.
127 Elias P, Williams ML, Maloney M, Fritsch P, Chung J-C: Applications of the diazacholesterol animal model of ichthyosis; in Marks R, Plewig G (eds): Skin Models. Berlin, Springer, 1986, pp 122–135.
128 Elias PM, Lampe MA, Chung JC, Williams ML: Diazacholesterol-induced ichthyosis in the hairless mouse. I. Morphologic, histochemical, and lipid biochemical characterization of a new animal model. Lab Invest 1983;48:565–577.
129 Feingold KR: The regulation and role of epidermal lipid synthesis. Adv Lipid Res 1991;24:57–82.
130 Cooper MK, Wassif CA, Krakowiak PA, et al: A defective response to hedgehog signaling in disorders of cholesterol biosynthesis. Nat Genet 2003; 33:508–513.
131 Clayton PT, Kalter DC, Atherton DJ, Besley GT, Broadhead DM: Peroxisomal enzyme deficiency in X-linked dominant Conradi-Hünermann syndrome. J Inherit Metab Dis 1989;12(suppl 2):358–360.
132 Holmes RD, Wilson GN, Hajra AK: Peroxisomal enzyme deficiency in the Conradi-Hünerman form of chondrodysplasia punctata. N Engl J Med 1987; 316:1608.
133 Wilson CJ, Aftimos S: X-linked dominant chondrodysplasia punctata: a peroxisomal disorder? Am J Med Genet 1998;78:300–302.
134 Goldyne ME, Williams ML: CHILD syndrome: phenotypic dichotomy in eicosanoid metabolism and proliferative rates among cultured dermal fibroblasts. J Clin Invest 1989;84:357–360.
135 Steinberg SJ, Dodt G, Raymond GV, Braverman NE, Moser AB, Moser HW: Peroxisome biogenesis disorders. Biochim Biophys Acta 2006;1763:1733–1748.
136 Liao H, Waters AJ, Goudie DR, et al: Filaggrin mutations are genetic modifying factors exacerbating X-linked ichthyosis. J Invest Dermatol 2007;127: 2795–2798.
137 Epstein EH Jr, Krauss RM, Shackleton CH: X-linked ichthyosis: increased blood cholesterol sulfate and electrophoretic mobility of low-density lipoprotein. Science 1981;214:659–660.
138 Bergner EA, Shapiro LJ: Metabolism of ^{3}H-dehydroepiandrosterone sulphate by subjects with steroid sulphatase deficiency. J Inherit Metab Dis 1988; 11:403–415.
139 Ibsen HH, Brandrup F, Secher B: Topical cholesterol treatment of recessive X-linked ichthyosis. Lancet 1984;ii:645.
140 Shapiro LJ: Steroid sulfatase deficiency and the genetics of the short arm of the human X chromosome. Adv Hum Genet 1985;14:331–381, 388–389.
141 Bradshaw KD, Carr BR: Placental sulfatase deficiency: maternal and fetal expression of steroid sulfatase deficiency and X-linked ichthyosis. Obstet Gynecol Surv 1986;41:401–413.

142 Lykkesfeldt G, Nielsen MD, Lykkesfeldt AE: Placental steroid sulfatase deficiency: biochemical diagnosis and clinical review. Obstet Gynecol 1984; 64:49–54.
143 David M, Israel N, Merksamer R, et al: Very low maternal serum unconjugated estriol and prenatal diagnosis of steroid sulfatase deficiency. Fetal Diagn Ther 1995;10:76–79.
144 Schoen E, Norem C, O'Keefe J, Krieger R, Walton D, To TT: Maternal serum unconjugated estriol as a predictor for Smith-Lemli-Opitz syndrome and other fetal conditions. Obstet Gynecol 2003;102:167–172.
145 Lykkesfeldt G, Hoyer H, Lykkesfeldt AE, Skakkebaek NE: Steroid sulphatase deficiency associated with testis cancer. Lancet 1983;ii:1456.
146 Koppe G, Marinkovic-Ilsen A, Rijken Y, De Groot WP, Jobsis AC: X-linked icthyosis: a sulphatase deficiency. Arch Dis Child 1978;53:803–806.
147 Webster D, France JT, Shapiro LJ, Weiss R: X-linked ichthyosis due to steroid-sulphatase deficiency. Lancet 1978;i:70–72.
148 Tiepolo L, Zuffardi O, Rodewald A: Nullisomy for the distal portion of Xp in a male child with a X/Y translocation. Hum Genet 1977;39:277–281.
149 Mohandas T, Shapiro LJ, Sparkes RS, Sparkes MC: Regional assignment of the steroid sulfatase-X-linked ichthyosis locus: implications for a noninactivated region on the short arm of human X chromosome. Proc Natl Acad Sci USA 1979;76:5779–5783.
150 Li XM, Yen P, Mohandas T, Shapiro LJ: A long range restriction map of the distal human X chromosome short arm around the steroid sulfatase locus. Nucleic Acids Res 1990;18:2783–2788.
151 Tiepolo L, Zuffardi O, Fraccaro M, et al: Assignment by deletion mapping of the steroid sulfatase X-linked ichthyosis locus to Xp223. Hum Genet 1980;54:205–206.
152 Ballabio A, Parenti G, Carrozzo R, et al: Isolation and characterization of a steroid sulfatase cDNA clone: genomic deletions in patients with X-chromosome-linked ichthyosis. Proc Natl Acad Sci USA 1987;84:4519–4523.
153 Bonifas JM, Morley BJ, Oakey RE, Kan YW, Epstein EH Jr: Cloning of a cDNA for steroid sulfatase: frequent occurrence of gene deletions in patients with recessive X chromosome-linked ichthyosis. Proc Natl Acad Sci USA 1987;84:9248–9251.
154 Conary JT, Lorkowski G, Schmidt B, et al: Genetic heterogeneity of steroid sulfatase deficiency revealed with cDNA for human steroid sulfatase. Biochem Biophys Res Commun 1987;144:1010–1017.
155 Gillard EF, Affara NA, Yates JR, et al: Deletion of a DNA sequence in eight of nine families with X-linked ichthyosis (steroid sulphatase deficiency). Nucleic Acids Res 1987;15:3977–3985.
156 Shapiro LJ, Yen P, Pomerantz D, Martin E, Rolewic L, Mohandas T: Molecular studies of deletions at the human steroid sulfatase locus. Proc Natl Acad Sci USA 1989;86:8477–8481.
157 Schmickel RD: Contiguous gene syndromes: a component of recognizable syndromes. J Pediatr 1986; 109:231–241.
158 Schnur RE, Trask BJ, van den Engh G, et al: An Xp22 microdeletion associated with ocular albinism and ichthyosis: approximation of breakpoints and estimation of deletion size by using cloned DNA probes and flow cytometry. Am J Hum Genet 1989; 45:706–720.
159 De Vries B, Eussen B, van Diggelen O, et al: Submicroscopic Xpter deletion in a boy with growth and mental retardation caused by a familial t(X;14). Am J Med Genet A 1999;87:189–194.
160 Willemsen R, Kroos M, Hoogeveen AT, et al: Ultrastructural localization of steroid sulphatase in cultured human fibroblasts by immunocytochemistry: a comparative study with lysosomal enzymes and the mannose 6-phosphate receptor. Histochem J 1988;20:41–51.
161 Dibbelt L, Herzog V, Kuss E: Human placental sterylsulfatase: immunocytochemical and biochemical localization. Biol Chem Hoppe Seyler 1989;370: 1093–1102.
162 Elias PM, Williams ML, Maloney ME, et al: Stratum corneum lipids in disorders of cornification: steroid sulfatase and cholesterol sulfate in normal desquamation and the pathogenesis of recessive X-linked ichthyosis. J Clin Invest 1984;74:1414–1421.
163 Epstein EH, Williams ML, Elias PM: The epidermal cholesterol sulfate cycle. J Am Acad Dermatol 1984; 10:866–868.
164 Long SA, Wertz PW, Strauss JS, Downing DT: Human stratum corneum polar lipids and desquamation. Arch Dermatol Res 1985;277:284–287.
165 Rearick JI, Albro PW, Jetten AM: Increase in cholesterol sulfotransferase activity during in vitro squamous differentiation of rabbit tracheal epithelial cells and its inhibition by retinoic acid. J Biol Chem 1987;262:13069–13074.
166 Rearick JI, Hesterberg TW, Jetten AM: Human bronchial epithelial cells synthesize cholesterol sulfate during squamous differentiation in vitro. J Cell Physiol 1987;133:573–578.
167 Rearick JI, Jetten AM: Accumulation of cholesterol 3-sulfate during in vitro squamous differentiation of rabbit tracheal epithelial cells and its regulation by retinoids. J Biol Chem 1986;261:13898–13904.

168 Jetten AM, George MA, Pettit GR, Herald CL, Rearick JI: Action of phorbol esters, bryostatins, and retinoic acid on cholesterol sulfate synthesis: relation to the multistep process of differentiation in human epidermal keratinocytes. J Invest Dermatol 1989;93:108–115.
169 Higashi Y, Fuda H, Yanai H, et al: Expression of cholesterol sulfotransferase (SULT2B1b) in human skin and primary cultures of human epidermal keratinocytes. J Invest Dermatol 2004;122:1207–1213.
170 Williams ML, Rutherford SL, Ponec M, Hincenbergs M, Placzek DR, Elias PM: Density-dependent variations in the lipid content and metabolism of cultured human keratinocytes. J Invest Dermatol 1988; 91:86–91.
171 Jetten AM, Brody AR, Deas MA, Hook GE, Rearick JI, Thacher SM: Retinoic acid and substratum regulate the differentiation of rabbit tracheal epithelial cells into squamous and secretory phenotype: morphological and biochemical characterization. Lab Invest 1987;56:654–664.
172 Kagehara M, Tachi M, Harii K, Iwamori M: Programmed expression of cholesterol sulfotransferase and transglutaminase during epidermal differentiation of murine skin development. Biochim Biophys Acta 1994;1215:183–189.
173 Hanley K, Jiang Y, Katagiri C, Feingold KR, Williams ML: Epidermal steroid sulfatase and cholesterol sulfotransferase are regulated during late gestation in the fetal rat. J Invest Dermatol 1997;108:871–875.
174 Komuves LG, Hanley K, Jiang Y, et al: Induction of selected lipid metabolic enzymes and differentiation-linked structural proteins by air exposure in fetal rat skin explants. J Invest Dermatol 1999;112: 303–309.
175 Jiang YJ, Kim P, Elias PM, Feingold KR: LXR and PPAR activators stimulate cholesterol sulfotransferase type 2 isoform 1b in human keratinocytes. J Lipid Res 2005;46:2657–2666.
176 Strott CA: Sulfonation and molecular action. Endocr Rev 2002;23:703–732.
177 Strott CA, Higashi Y: Cholesterol sulfate in human physiology: what's it all about? J Lipid Res 2003;44: 1268–1278.
178 Kashiwagi M, Ohba M, Chida K, Kuroki T: Protein kinase C eta (PKC eta): its involvement in keratinocyte differentiation. J Biochem (Tokyo) 2002;132: 853–857.
179 Denning MF, Dlugosz AA, Williams EK, Szallasi Z, Blumberg PM, Yuspa SH: Specific protein kinase C isozymes mediate the induction of keratinocyte differentiation markers by calcium. Cell Growth Differ 1995;6:149–157.
180 Ikuta T, Chida K, Tajima O, et al: Cholesterol sulfate, a novel activator for the eta isoform of protein kinase C. Cell Growth Differ 1994;5:943–947.
181 Kuroki T, Ikuta T, Kashiwagi M, et al: Cholesterol sulfate, an activator of protein kinase C mediating squamous cell differentiation: a review. Mutat Res 2000;462:189–195.
182 Kawabe S, Ikuta T, Ohba M, et al: Cholesterol sulfate activates transcription of transglutaminase 1 gene in normal human keratinocytes. J Invest Dermatol 1998;111:1098–1102.
183 Hanley K, Wood L, Ng DC, et al: Cholesterol sulfate stimulates involucrin transcription in keratinocytes by increasing Fra-1, Fra-2, and Jun D. J Lipid Res 2001;42:390–398.
184 Kubilus J, Tarascio AJ, Baden HP: Steroid-sulfatase deficiency in sex-linked ichthyosis. Am J Hum Genet 1979;31:50–53.
185 Williams ML, Elias PM: Stratum corneum lipids in disorders of cornification: increased cholesterol sulfate content of stratum corneum in recessive X-linked ichthyosis. J Clin Invest 1981;68:1404–1410.
186 Ranasinghe AW, Wertz PW, Downing DT, Mackenzie IC: Lipid composition of cohesive and desquamated corneocytes from mouse ear skin. J Invest Dermatol 1986;86:187–190.
187 Grayson S, Johnson-Winegar AG, Wintroub BU, Isseroff RR, Epstein EH Jr, Elias PM: Lamellar body-enriched fractions from neonatal mice: preparative techniques and partial characterization. J Invest Dermatol 1985;85:289–294.
188 Ponec M, Williams ML: Cholesterol sulfate uptake and outflux in cultured human keratinocytes. Arch Dermatol Res 1986;279:32–36.
189 Lavrijsen AP, Oestmann E, Hermans J, Boddé HE, Vermeer BJ, Ponec M: Barrier function parameters in various keratinization disorders: transepidermal water loss and vascular response to hexyl nicotinate. Br J Dermatol 1993;129:547–553.
190 Johansen JD, Ramsing D, Vejlsgaard G, Agner T: Skin barrier properties in patients with recessive X-linked ichthyosis. Acta Derm Venereol 1995;75: 202–204.
191 Zettersten E, Man MQ, Sato J, et al: Recessive X-linked ichthyosis: role of cholesterol-sulfate accumulation in the barrier abnormality. J Invest Dermatol 1998;111:784–790.
192 Feingold KR, Man MQ, Menon GK, Cho SS, Brown BE, Elias PM: Cholesterol synthesis is required for cutaneous barrier function in mice. J Clin Invest 1990;86:1738–1745.
193 Williams ML, Rutherford SL, Feingold KR: Effects of cholesterol sulfate on lipid metabolism in cultured human keratinocytes and fibroblasts. J Lipid Res 1987;28:955–967.
194 Frost P, Weinstein GD, Van Scott EJ: The ichthyosiform dermatoses. II. Autoradiographic studies of epidermal proliferation. J Invest Dermatol 1966;47: 561–567.

195 Ekholm IE, Brattsand M, Egelrud T: Stratum corneum tryptic enzyme in normal epidermis: a missing link in the desquamation process? J Invest Dermatol 2000;114:56–63.
196 Sato J, Denda M, Nakanishi J, Nomura J, Koyama J: Cholesterol sulfate inhibits proteases that are involved in desquamation of stratum corneum. J Invest Dermatol 1998;111:189–193.
197 Williams ML: Lipids in normal and pathological desquamation. Adv Lipid Res 1991;24:211–262.
198 Hachem JP, Crumrine D, Fluhr J, Brown BE, Feingold KR, Elias PM: pH directly regulates epidermal permeability barrier homeostasis, and stratum corneum integrity/cohesion. J Invest Dermatol 2003;121:345–353.
199 Hachem JP, Fowler A, Behne M, Fluhr J, Feingold K, Elias P: Increased stratum corneum pH promotes activation and release of primary cytokines from the stratum corneum attributable to activation of serine proteases. J Invest Dermatol 2002;119:258.
200 Hachem JP, Roelandt T, Schurer N, et al: Acute acidification of stratum corneum membrane domains using polyhydroxyl acids improves lipid processing and inhibits degradation of corneodesmosomes. J Invest Dermatol 20010;130:500–510.
201 Ohman H, Vahlquist A: The pH gradient over the stratum corneum differs in X-linked recessive and autosomal dominant ichthyosis: a clue to the molecular origin of the 'acid skin mantle'? J Invest Dermatol 1998;111:674–677.
202 Abraham W, Wertz PW, Landmann L, Downing DT: Stratum corneum lipid liposomes: calcium-induced transformation into lamellar sheets. J Invest Dermatol 1987;88:212–214.
203 Hatfield RM, Fung LW: A new model system for lipid interactions in stratum corneum vesicles: effects of lipid composition, calcium, and pH. Biochemistry 1999;38:784–791.
204 Sidransky E: Gaucher disease: complexity in a 'simple' disorder. Mol Genet Metab 2004;83:6–15.
205 Sidransky E, Fartasch M, Lee RE, et al: Epidermal abnormalities may distinguish type 2 from type 1 and type 3 of Gaucher disease. Pediatr Res 1996;39: 134–141.
206 Stone DL, Carey WF, Christodoulou J, et al: Type 2 Gaucher disease: the collodion baby phenotype revisited. Arch Dis Child Fetal Neonatal Ed 2000; 82:F163–F166.
207 Holleran WM, Takagi Y, Menon GK, Legler G, Feingold KR, Elias PM: Processing of epidermal glucosylceramides is required for optimal mammalian cutaneous permeability barrier function. J Clin Invest 1993;91:1656–1664.
208 Schmuth M, Man MQ, Weber F, et al: Permeability barrier disorder in Niemann-Pick disease: sphingomyelin-ceramide processing required for normal barrier homeostasis. J Invest Dermatol 2000;115: 459–466.
209 Schmuth M, Weber F, Paschke E, Sepp N, Fritsch P: Delayed epidermal permeability repair in patients with sphingomyelinase deficiency (Niemann-Pick disease). J Invest Dermatol 1999;112:542.
210 Uchida Y, Hara M, Nishio H, et al: Epidermal sphingomyelins are precursors for selected stratum corneum ceramides. J Lipid Res 2000;41:2071–2082.
211 Holleran WM, Man MQ, Gao WN, Menon GK, Elias PM, Feingold KR: Sphingolipids are required for mammalian epidermal barrier function: inhibition of sphingolipid synthesis delays barrier recovery after acute perturbation. J Clin Invest 1991;88: 1338–1345.
212 Holleran WM, Ginns EI, Menon GK, et al: Consequences of beta-glucocerebrosidase deficiency in epidermis: ultrastructure and permeability barrier alterations in Gaucher disease. J Clin Invest 1994;93: 1756–1764.
213 Jensen JM, Schutze S, Forl M, Kronke M, Proksch E: Roles for tumor necrosis factor receptor p55 and sphingomyelinase in repairing the cutaneous permeability barrier. J Clin Invest 1999;104:1761–1770.
214 Marsh NL, Elias PM, Holleran WM: Glucosylceramides stimulate murine epidermal hyperproliferation. J Clin Invest 1995;95:2903–2909.
215 Milger K, Herrmann T, Becker C, et al: Cellular uptake of fatty acids driven by the ER-localized acyl-CoA synthetase FATP4. J Cell Sci 2006;119: 4678–4688.
216 Harris IR, Farrell AM, Memon RA, Grunfeld C, Elias PM, Feingold KR: Expression and regulation of mRNA for putative fatty acid transport related proteins and fatty acyl CoA synthase in murine epidermis and cultured human keratinocytes. J Invest Dermatol 1998;111:722–726.
217 Schmuth M, Ortegon AM, Mao-Qiang M, Elias PM, Feingold KR, Stahl A: Differential expression of fatty acid transport proteins in epidermis and skin appendages. J Invest Dermatol 2005;125:1174–1181.
218 Jia Z, Moulson CL, Pei Z, Miner JH, Watkins PA: Fatty acid transport protein 4 is the principal very long chain fatty acyl-CoA synthetase in skin fibroblasts. J Biol Chem 2007;282:20573–20583.
219 Ziboh VA, Chapkin RS: Metabolism and function of skin lipids. Prog Lipid Res 1988;27:81–105.
220 Anton-Lamprecht I: Diagnostic ultrastructure of non-neoplastic diseases; in Papadimitriou J, Spagnolo D (eds): The Skin. Edinburgh, Churchill Livingstone, 1992, pp 459–550.

221 Williams ML, Elias PM: From basketweave to barrier: unifying concepts for the pathogenesis of the disorders of cornification. Arch Dermatol 1993;129: 626–629.
222 Akiyama M: The pathogenesis of severe congenital ichthyosis of the neonate. J Dermatol Sci 1999;21:96–104.
223 Williams ML, Elias PM: Genetically transmitted, generalized disorders of cornification – the ichthyoses. Dermatol Clin 1987;5:155–178.
224 Nussey DH, Postma E, Glenapp P, Visser ME: Selection on heritable phenotypic plasticity in a wild bird population. Science 2005;310:304–306.
225 Akiyama M, Sugiyama-Nakagiri Y, Sakai K, et al: Mutations in lipid transporter ABCA12 in harlequin ichthyosis and functional recovery by corrective gene transfer. J Clin Invest 2005;115:1777–1784.
226 Kelsell DP, Norgett EE, Unsworth H, et al: Mutations in ABCA12 underlie the severe congenital skin disease harlequin ichthyosis. Am J Hum Genet 2005; 76:794–803.
227 Sakai K, Akiyama M, Sugiyama-Nakagiri Y, McMillan JR, Sawamura D, Shimizu H: Localization of ABCA12 from Golgi apparatus to lamellar granules in human upper epidermal keratinocytes. Exp Dermatol 2007;16:920–926.
228 Hollenstein K, Frei D, Locher K: Structure of an ABC transporter in complex with its binding protein. Nature 2007;446:213–216.
229 Allikmets R, Gerrard B, Hutchinson A, Dean M: Characterization of the human ABC superfamily: isolation and mapping of 21 new genes using the expressed sequence tags database. Hum Mol Genet 1996;5:1649–1655.
230 Borst P, Elferink RO: Mammalian ABC transporters in health and disease. Annu Rev Biochem 2002;71: 537–592.
231 Dean M, Rzhetsky A, Allikmets R: The human ATP-binding cassette (ABC) transporter superfamily. Genome Res 2001;11:1156–1166.
232 Jiang YJ, Lu B, Kim P, et al: PPAR and LXR activators regulate ABCA12 expression in human keratinocytes. J Invest Dermatol 2008;128:104–109.
233 Thomas AC, Cullup T, Norgett EE, et al: ABCA12 is the major harlequin ichthyosis gene. J Invest Dermatol 2006;126:2408–2413.
234 Elias PM, Fartasch M, Crumrine D, Behne M, Uchida Y, Holleran WM: Origin of the corneocyte lipid envelope (CLE): observations in harlequin ichthyosis and cultured human keratinocytes. J Invest Dermatol 2000;115:765–769.
235 Yamanaka Y, Akiyama M, Sugiyama-Nakagiri Y, et al: Expression of the keratinocyte lipid transporter ABCA12 in developing and reconstituted human epidermis. Am J Pathol 2007;171:43–52.
236 Dale BA, Holbrook KA, Fleckman P, Kimball JR, Brumbaugh S, Sybert VP: Heterogeneity in harlequin ichthyosis, an inborn error of epidermal keratinization: variable morphology and structural protein expression and a defect in lamellar granules. J Invest Dermatol 1990;94:6–18.
237 Milner ME, O'Guin WM, Holbrook KA, Dale BA: Abnormal lamellar granules in harlequin ichthyosis. J Invest Dermatol 1992;99:824–829.
238 Uchida Y, Holleran WM, Elias PM: On the effects of topical synthetic pseudoceramides: comparison of possible keratinocyte toxicities provoked by the pseudoceramides, PC104 and BIO391, and natural ceramides. J Dermatol Sci 2008;51:37–43.
239 Choate KA, Williams ML, Elias PM, Khavari PA: Transglutaminase 1 expression in a patient with features of harlequin ichthyosis: case report. J Am Acad Dermatol 1998;38:325–329.
240 Rassner UA, Crumrine DA, Nau P, Elias PM: Microwave incubation improves lipolytic enzyme preservation for ultrastructural cytochemistry. Histochem J 1997;29:387–392.
241 Brattsand M, Stefansson K, Lundh C, Haasum Y, Egelrud T: A proteolytic cascade of kallikreins in the stratum corneum. J Invest Dermatol 2005;124: 198–203.
242 Caubet C, Jonca N, Brattsand M, et al: Degradation of corneodesmosome proteins by two serine proteases of the kallikrein family, SCTE/KLK5/hK5 and SCCE/KLK7/hK7. J Invest Dermatol 2004;122:1235–1244.
243 Horikoshi T, Igarashi S, Uchiwa H, Brysk H, Brysk MM: Role of endogenous cathepsin D-like and chymotrypsin-like proteolysis in human epidermal desquamation. Br J Dermatol 1999;141:453–459.
244 Zeeuwen PL: Epidermal differentiation: the role of proteases and their inhibitors. Eur J Cell Biol 2004; 83:761–773.
245 Sprecher E, Ishida-Yamamoto A, Mizrahi-Koren M, et al: A mutation in *SNAP29*, coding for a SNARE protein involved in intracellular trafficking, causes a novel neurocutaneous syndrome characterized by cerebral dysgenesis, neuropathy, ichthyosis, and palmoplantar keratoderma. Am J Hum Genet 2005; 77:242–251.
246 Saba TG, Montpetit A, Verner A, et al: An atypical form of erythrokeratodermia variabilis maps to chromosome 7q22. Hum Genet 2005;116:167–171.
247 Montpetit A, Cote S, Brustein E, et al: Disruption of AP1S1, causing a novel neurocutaneous syndrome, perturbs development of the skin and spinal cord. PLoS Genet 2008;4:e1000296.

248 Gissen P, Johnson CA, Morgan NV, et al: Mutations in *VPS33B,* encoding a regulator of SNARE-dependent membrane fusion, cause arthrogryposis-renal dysfunction-cholestasis (ARC) syndrome. Nat Genet 2004;36:400–404.

249 Hershkovitz D, Mandel H, Ishida-Yamamoto A, et al: Defective lamellar granule secretion in arthrogryposis, renal dysfunction, and cholestasis syndrome caused by a mutation in VPS33B. Arch Dermatol 2008;144:334–340.

250 Gissen P, Tee L, Johnson CA, et al: Clinical and molecular genetic features of ARC syndrome. Hum Genet 2006;120:396–409.

251 Coleman RA, Van Hove JL, Morris CR, Rhoads JM, Summar ML: Cerebral defects and nephrogenic diabetes insipidus with the ARC syndrome: additional findings or a new syndrome (ARCC-NDI)? Am J Med Genet 1997;72:335–338.

252 Deal JE, Barratt TM, Dillon MJ: Fanconi syndrome, ichthyosis, dysmorphism, jaundice and diarrhoea – a new syndrome. Pediatr Nephrol 1990;4:308–313.

253 Eastham KM, McKiernan PJ, Milford DV, et al: ARC syndrome: an expanding range of phenotypes. Arch Dis Child 2001;85:415–420.

254 Elias PM, Cullander C, Mauro T, et al: The secretory granular cell: the outermost granular cell as a specialized secretory cell. J Invest Dermatol Symp Proc 1998;3:87–100.

255 Gonelle-Gispert C, Molinete M, Halban PA, Sadoul K: Membrane localization and biological activity of SNAP-25 cysteine mutants in insulin-secreting cells. J Cell Sci 2000;113:3197–3205.

256 Feng D, Crane K, Rozenvayn N, Dvorak AM, Flaumenhaft R: Subcellular distribution of 3 functional platelet SNARE proteins: human cellubrevin, SNAP-23, and syntaxin 2. Blood 2002;99:4006–4014.

257 Steegmaier M, Yang B, Yoo JS, et al: Three novel proteins of the syntaxin/SNAP-25 family. J Biol Chem 1998;273:34171–34179.

258 Ugur O, Jones TL: A proline-rich region and nearby cysteine residues target XLalphas to the Golgi complex region. Mol Biol Cell 2000;11:1421–1432.

259 Hohenstein AC, Roche PA: SNAP-29 is a promiscuous syntaxin-binding SNARE. Biochem Biophys Res Commun 2001;285:167–171.

260 Wong SH, Xu Y, Zhang T, et al: GS32, a novel Golgi SNARE of 32 kDa, interacts preferentially with syntaxin 6. Mol Biol Cell 1999;10:119–134.

261 Hepp R, Langley K: SNAREs during development. Cell Tissue Res 2001;305:247–253.

Chapter 3

Inherited Disorders of Accelerated Desquamation

3.1. Netherton Syndrome

3.1.1 Clinical Characteristics and Biochemical Genetics of Netherton Syndrome

Patients with Netherton syndrome (NS, ichthyosis linearis circumflexa, Comèl-Netherton syndrome; OMIM No. 256500) display generalized scaling with marked inflammation that clinically resembles severe atopic dermatitis (AD) [1–3]. Skin disease is usually evident at (or shortly after) birth, typically presenting with a generalized erythroderma and scaling, which can be confused with psoriasis, particularly in infants [4]. Although histological analysis shows epidermal hyperplasia, as in psoriasis, a thin (rather than thick), parakeratotic stratum corneum is present [4]. Although the rash does not improve over time, in older children and adults with NS, a unique scaling pattern, termed ichthyosis linearis circumflexa, may develop in which serpiginous areas of 'double-edged' scales are present. Patients also experience severe pruritus, temperature instability and low sweat secretion. Atopy with anaphylactic reactions to food allergens, high serum IgE levels, eosinophilia and asthma are additional, common features of NS [1–3].

The high mortality of NS in the first year of life is due to electrolyte imbalance, dehydration, failure to thrive (severe growth failure) and/or systemic infections (see below). Growth failure can be attributed specifically to the severe permeability barrier defect which results in excessive loss of calories through heat of evaporation [5, 6] [chapter 1, this vol., pp. 1–29]. As a result of the severe permeability barrier abnormality, patients with NS are also at risk for excessive systemic absorption of topical medications [7, 8].

The skin changes are typically accompanied by hair shaft abnormalities, including short or thin hair, patchy, very slowly growing eyelashes and a pathognomonic hair shaft defect, called trichorrhexis invaginata or 'bamboo hair', in which the distal hair segment telescopes onto the proximal hair shaft [9]. Yet, only a minority of hairs may display this defect; trichorrhexis invaginata may only appear over time [10], and finally some genotyped NS patients appear to lack hair abnormalities [G. Richard, pers. commun.]. Since a negative hair mount does not rule out NS, NS can masquerade as severe AD or infantile psoriasis.

As noted above, systemic infections are a significant cause of mortality in NS. Patients are at increased risk for severe viral skin infections, such as herpes simplex and human papillomavirus. Moreover, cases of human-papillomavirus-associated, nonmelanoma skin cancer have been reported [11–15]. Both cutaneous and, in infants, systemic infections could result from a proteolytic attack on epidermal antimicrobial peptides, particularly the cathelicidin carboxy fragment LL-37. Indeed, disturbed cathelicidin proteolysis has been linked to lymphoepithelial Kazal-type 5 inhibitor (LEKTI) deficiency in an NS mouse model [16]. Yet, these abnormalities in antimicrobial defense could also reflect in part Th2-mediated downregulation of certain antimicrobial peptides, including LL-37, as occurs in AD [17].

3.1.2 Biochemical Genetics

NS is most frequently caused by recessive, and in a minority of cases single-allele (<20%), loss-of-function mutations in the serine protease inhibitor Kazal-type 5 gene *(SPINK5)* [9]. *SPINK5* encodes for the serine protease inhibitor LEKTI-1 [1, 18–20]. A large number of stop codon, splice site, frameshift and missense mutations has been described which result in either absent or reduced inhibitor levels [9, 20–22; G. Richard, pers. commun.]. The severity of the hair shaft abnormality appears to be independent of the type of mutations in NS [G. Richard, pers. commun.].

While LEKTI-1 is expressed in skin, mucous membranes, tonsils and thymus [19, 23], epidermis expression is restricted to both the granular layer, where it localizes to a discrete subset of lamellar bodies [24], and to the stratum corneum interstices [25]. LEKTI-1 is normally cleaved into 15 active domains that suppress serine protease (kallikrein) activity. The likely, specific biological targets of LEKTI-1 include both the stratum corneum trypsin- and chymotrypsin-like enzymes (kallikrein 5 and 7, respectively) [26–29], which degrade corneodesmosome E-cadherins [30]. LEKTI-1 deficiency, in turn, results in largely unopposed, serine protease activity in NS [25]. A nearby gene, *SPINK9*, encodes the closely related LEKTI-2, which localizes primarily to the epidermis of palms and soles [31, 32]. While LEKTI-2 inhibits kallikrein 5, and therefore could regulate desquamation from the palms and soles [31, 32], in contrast to LEKTI-1, it also exhibits potent antimicrobial activity [33].

3.1.3 Pathogenesis of Netherton Syndrome

Our laboratory has shown that the extent of residual LEKTI-1 protein expression correlates inversely with total residual serine protease activity, and that in moderate-

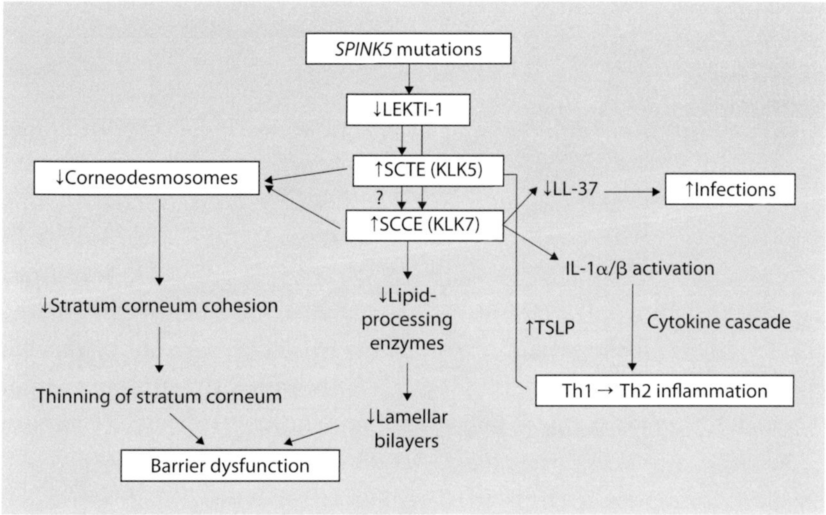

Fig. 1. Pathogenesis of NS. SCTE = Stratum corneum tryptic enzyme; SCCE = stratum corneum chymotryptic enzyme; KLK = kallikrein; TSLP = thymocyte-stimulating lymphopoietin.

to-severe cases, protease activity extends deeper into the nucleated epidermal layers than in milder cases [25]. Although we did not determine whether milder cases represent single-allele or missense mutations, Sprecher et al. [9] showed that the genetic abnormality correlates with the phenotype. Defective serine protease inhibitor activity, in turn, results in premature corneodesmosome degradation, accounting for both thinning of the stratum corneum and inactivation of lipid hydrolases required for processing of secreted lamellar body lipids into the nonpolar species that form the lamellar bilayers [25]. Thus, LEKTI-1 plays a key role in both barrier function and in the restriction of corneocyte desquamation in normal skin, as demonstrated by the severe permeability/desquamation abnormalities in NS.

LEKTI-1 deficiency also favors the development of inflammation, not only by activating the cytokine cascade [chapter 1, this vol., pp. 1–29], but also by initiating Th2 inflammation (fig. 1). Unrestricted kallikrein 5 activates proteinase-activated receptor 2, which in turn stimulates nuclear-factor-κB-mediated overexpression of thymocyte-stimulating lymphopoietin, intercellular adhesion molecule 1, tumor necrosis factor α and IL-8 [34].

While loss-of-function *SPINK5* mutations in transgenic knockout mice result in early postpartum death [35], most humans with NS survive the perinatal period, due to both compensatory, suprabasal upregulation of desmosomal proteins and accelerated lamellar body secretion [25, 36]. Nevertheless, the secreted contents of lamellar bodies are incompletely processed into functional lamellar bilayers in NS due to unchecked proteolytic degradation of lipid-processing enzymes [25] (fig. 1).

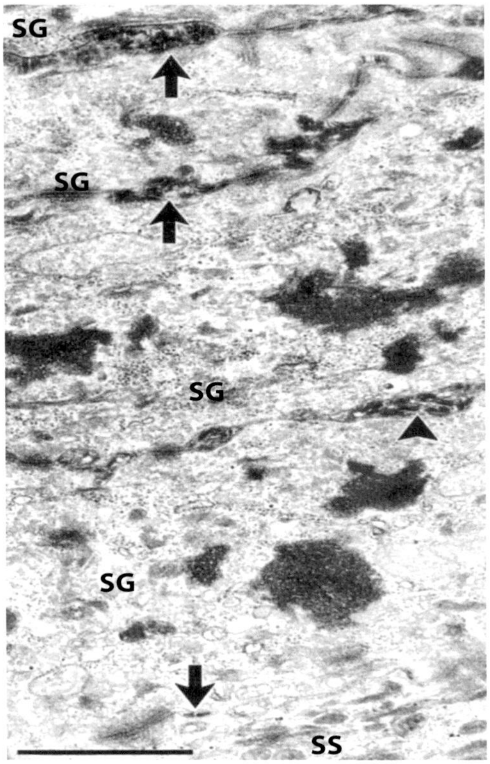

Fig. 2. Premature lamellar body secretion in NS. Secreted lamellar body contents are found in the intercellular spaces (arrows and arrowhead) of the nucleated layers. SG = Stratum granulosum; SS = stratum spinosum (modified from Fartasch et al. [36]). Magnification bar = 1 μm.

3.1.4 Cellular Pathogenesis and Diagnostic Ultrastructure

On routine electron microscopy, multilocular, extracellular vesicles have been described at the level of the stratum spinosum and stratum granulosum [37–40]. Closer examination reveals these vesicles to comprise the contents of prematurely secreted lamellar bodies [36] (fig. 2). Yet, while premature secretion of lamellar body contents is a distinctive feature of NS, it is not diagnostic, since this feature can also occur in other hyperproliferative disorders, such as psoriasis.

Overall, stratum corneum thickness is markedly reduced in NS [41] due to accelerated proteolysis of corneodesmosomes [25]. Thus, while NS is a 'true' disorder of cornification, it is not a 'true' ichthyosis. Excess protease activity in NS also explains both the reduced quantities of lamellar bilayers [25] and their highly abnormal morphology (fig. 3) [5, 25, 36]. The few membrane structures that persist display evidence of delayed membrane maturation, again likely reflecting accelerated destruction of lipid-processing enzymes by excess serine protease activity [25].

The key ultrastructural features of NS include: (1) a thin, loosely cohesive stratum corneum due to premature degradation of corneodesmosomes; (2) premature

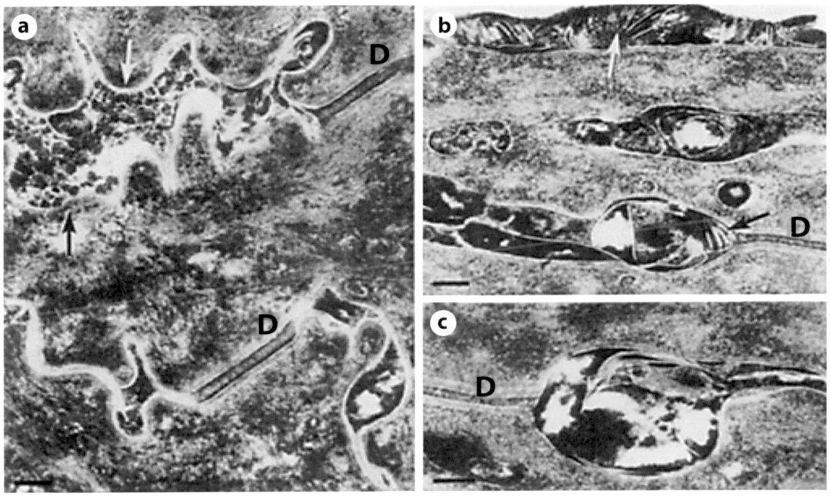

Fig. 3. Decreased and abnormal lamellar bilayers in NS; D = corneodesmosomes (modified from Fartasch et al. [36]). Magnification bars = 1 μm. **a** Lamellar lipid bilayers separated by granular, electron-dense material in upper regions of the stratum corneum. **b**, **c** Decreased lamellar membranes, which are interspersed with amorphous electron-dense material (arrows).

secretion of normal-appearing lamellar bodies between several nucleated cell layers beneath the stratum corneum, and (3) a paucity of extracellular lamellar bilayers, which are disorganized and display an 'immature' (unprocessed) appearance (fig. 4). Although none of these features alone is diagnostic, this triad together is sufficiently characteristic to strongly suggest the diagnosis of NS.

3.2. Relationship of Netherton Syndrome to Atopic Dermatitis

NS often presents as severe AD with elevated IgE levels, mucosal atopy and anaphylactic food reactions (see above); hence, an exploration of pathogenic mechanisms in NS may provide insights into AD pathogenesis (fig. 5). Diminished LEKTI-1 activity in NS likely also leads to cutaneous inflammation, because serine proteases activate IL-1α/β in corneocytes [42], initiating the 'cytokine cascade' [43], and a serine protease (i.e. kallikrein 5) can activate Th2 cytokines, independent of allergen exposure [34]. In some population studies, polymorphisms in the *SPINK5* gene (missense variants) are also associated with AD and mucosal atopy [44]. Moreover, it has recently been proposed that an acquired deficiency of LEKTI-1, due to proteolytic consumption of the inhibitor, could also contribute to the pathogenesis of AD [33]. In the next chapter [this vol., pp. 98–127], we provide further details about the link between AD and ichthyosis vulgaris, also briefly summarized in figure 5.

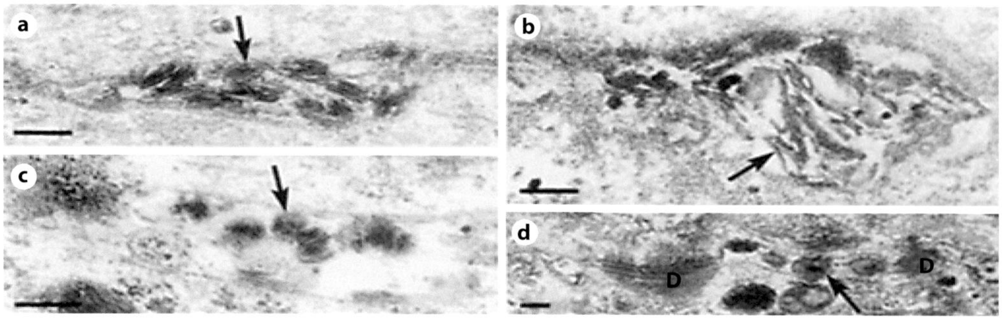

Fig. 4. Delayed membrane maturation in NS (modified from Fartasch et al. [36]). Magnification bars = 1 μm. **a–c** Arrows reveal unprocessed secreted lamellar-body-derived lipids, as foreshortened lamellar membranes in intercellular spaces. **d** Extruded lamellar body lipids do not disperse normally at the stratum granulosum/stratum corneum interface. Very few corneodesmosomes (D) remain in the lower stratum corneum.

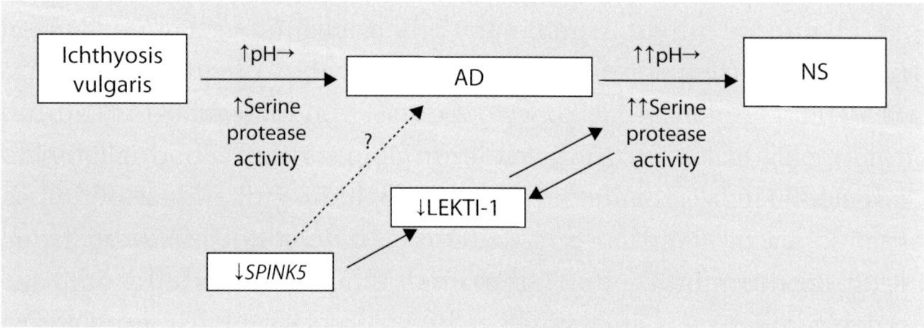

Fig. 5. Relationship of NS to AD and ichthyosis vulgaris.

3.3. Peeling Skin Syndrome

Peeling skin syndrome (PSS) type B (OMIM No. 270300) is a recessively inherited disorder, characterized by continuous skin peeling and variable erythroderma, with clinical features that overlap with mild NS. PSS is rare and most often reported in consanguineous families of Middle Eastern origin [1, 45]. Following a neonatal onset, patients display lifelong peeling of the stratum corneum, with or without an underlying erythroderma. PSS type A (OMIM No. 609796) is typically noninflammatory, asymptomatic and characterized by generalized scales of different sizes and shapes [1]. PSS type A typically localizes to the distal extremities ('acral PSS') or to the face [46, 47]. These localized PSS variants have been associated with loss-of-function mutations in transglutaminase 5 [48, 49], 1 of 3 transglutaminase genes (along with *TGM1* and *TGM3*) that mediate cross-linking of corneocyte envelope precursors [50]. In contrast, PSS type B patients present with a low-grade congenital ichthyosiform erythroderma phenotype, with migratory patches of scaling and atopic features, including pruritus and elevated serum IgE levels, consistent with mild NS. Although, *SPINK5* mutations have been reported in some PSS type B patients [51], despite evidence of increased serine protease activity, no *SPINK5* mutations have yet been identified in other PSS type B patients [52]. Recently, PSS type B has been linked to mutations in the corneodesmosome protein, corneodesmosin [53].

The histology and ultrastructure of PSS type A is characteristic: psoriasiform hyperplasia with corneocytes separating from one another just above the granular cell layer, as well as variable extracellular deposits of an unknown nature [54], and localized variants can show the same ultrastructural features [55]. In PSS type B, the cleavage plane can extend further downward into the granular cell layer [56]. Thus, decreased cohesion of corneocytes is a shared feature of both NS and PSS type B, which likely explains their overlapping clinical features. Whether other features of NS are present is not yet known, because RuO_4 postfixation has not yet been utilized to assess disease pathogenesis.

3.4. References

1 Traupe H: Ichthyosis: A Guide to Clinical Diagnosis, Genetic Counseling, and Therapy. New York, Springer, 1989, p 253.

2 Judge MR, Morgan G, Harper JI: A clinical and immunological study of Netherton's syndrome. Br J Dermatol 1994;131:615–621.

3 Griffiths W, Judge M, Leigh I: Disorders of keratinization; in Champion R, et al (eds): Textbook of Dermatology. Oxford, Blackwell Science, 1998, pp 1486–1488.

4 Oji V, Tadini G, Akiyama M, et al: Revised nomenclature and classification of inherited ichthyoses: results of the first ichthyosis consensus conference in Sorèze 2009. J Am Acad Dermatol 2010, Epub, ahead of print.

5 Moskowitz DG, Fowler AJ, Heyman MB, et al: Pathophysiologic basis for growth failure in children with ichthyosis: an evaluation of cutaneous ultrastructure, epidermal permeability barrier function, and energy expenditure. J Pediatr 2004;145:82–92.

6 Fowler AJ, Moskowitz DG, Wong A, Cohen SP, Williams ML, Heyman MB: Nutritional status and gastrointestinal structure and function in children with ichthyosis and growth failure. J Pediatr Gastroenterol Nutr 2004;38:164–169.

7 Allen A, Siegfried E, Silverman R, et al: Significant absorption of topical tacrolimus in 3 patients with Netherton syndrome. Arch Dermatol 2001;137:747–750.

8 Smith DL, Smith JG, Wong SW, de Shazo RD: Netherton's syndrome: a syndrome of elevated IgE and characteristic skin and hair findings. J Allergy Clin Immunol 1995;95:116–123.

9 Sprecher E, Chavanas S, Di Giovanna JJ, et al: The spectrum of pathogenic mutations in *SPINK5* in 19 families with Netherton syndrome: implications for mutation detection and first case of prenatal diagnosis. J Invest Dermatol 2001;117:179–187.

10 Richard G: Disorders of cornification; in Sprecher E (ed): Progress in Monogenic Hair Disorders. New York, Nova Biomedical, 2006, pp 153–196.

11 Saghari S, Woolery-Lloyd H, Nouri K: Squamous cell carcinoma in a patient with Netherton's syndrome. Int J Dermatol 2002;41:415–416.

12 Kubler HC, Kuhn W, Rummel HH, Kaufmann I, Kaufmann M: Development of cancer (vulvar cancer) in the Netherton syndrome (ichthyosis, hair anomalies, atopic diathesis (in German). Geburtshilfe Frauenheilkd 1987;47:742–744.

13 Hintner H, Jaschke E, Fritsch P: Netherton syndrome: weakened immunity, generalized verrucosis and carcinogenesis (in German). Hautarzt 1980;31: 428–432.

14 Krasagakis K, Ioannidou DJ, Stephanidou M, Manios A, Panayiotides JG, Tosca AD: Early development of multiple epithelial neoplasms in Netherton syndrome. Dermatology 2003;207:182–184.

15 Weber F, Fuchs PG, Pfister HJ, Hintner H, Fritsch P, Hoepfl R: Human papillomavirus infection in Netherton's syndrome. Br J Dermatol 2001;144:1044–1049.

16 Yamasaki K, Schauber J, Coda A, et al: Kallikrein-mediated proteolysis regulates the antimicrobial effects of cathelicidins in skin. Faseb J 2006;20:2068–2080.

17 Ong PY, Ohtake T, Brandt C, et al: Endogenous antimicrobial peptides and skin infections in atopic dermatitis. N Engl J Med 2002;347:1151–1160.

18 Wile U: Familial study of three unusual cases of congenital ichthyosiform erythroderma. Arch Dermatol Syphilol 1924;10:487–498.

19 Magert HJ, Standker L, Kreutzmann P, et al: LEKTI, a novel 15-domain type of human serine proteinase inhibitor. J Biol Chem 1999;274:21499–21502.

20 Chavanas S, Bodemer C, Rochat A, et al: Mutations in *SPINK5,* encoding a serine protease inhibitor, cause Netherton syndrome. Nat Genet 2000;25:141–142.

21 Bitoun E, Chavanas S, Irvine AD, et al: Netherton syndrome: disease expression and spectrum of *SPINK5* mutations in 21 families. J Invest Dermatol 2002;118:352–361.

22 Raghunath M, Tontsidou L, Oji V, et al: *SPINK5* and Netherton syndrome: novel mutations, demonstration of missing LEKTI, and differential expression of transglutaminases. J Invest Dermatol 2004;123:474–483.

23 Walden M, Kreutzmann P, Drögemüller K, John H, Forssmann WG, Mägert H-J: Biochemical features, molecular biology and clinical relevance of the human 15-domain serine proteinase inhibitor LEKTI. Biol Chem 2002;383:1139–1141.

24 Ishida-Yamamoto A, Deraison C, Bonnart C, et al: LEKTI is localized in lamellar granules, separated from KLK5 and KLK7, and is secreted in the extracellular spaces of the superficial stratum granulosum. J Invest Dermatol 2005;124:360–366.

25 Hachem JP, Wagberg F, Schmuth M, et al: Serine protease activity and residual LEKTI expression determine phenotype in Netherton syndrome. J Invest Dermatol 2006;126:1609–1621.

26 Egelrud T, Brattsand M, Kreutzmann P, et al: hK5 and hK7, two serine proteinases abundant in human skin, are inhibited by LEKTI domain 6. Br J Dermatol 2005;153:1200–1203.

27 Caubet C, Jonca N, Brattsand M, et al: Degradation of corneodesmosome proteins by two serine proteases of the kallikrein family, SCTE/KLK5/hK5 and SCCE/KLK7/hK7. J Invest Dermatol 2004;122:1235–1244.

28 Borgono CA, Michael IP, Komatsu N, et al: A potential role for multiple tissue kallikrein serine proteases in epidermal desquamation. J Biol Chem 2007;282:3640–3652.

29 Schechter NM, Choi EJ, Wang ZM, et al: Inhibition of human kallikreins 5 and 7 by the serine protease inhibitor lympho-epithelial Kazal-type inhibitor (LEKTI). Biol Chem 2005;386:1173–1184.

30 Descargues P, Deraison C, Prost C, et al: Corneodesmosomal cadherins are preferential targets of stratum corneum trypsin- and chymotrypsin-like hyperactivity in Netherton syndrome. J Invest Dermatol 2006;126:1622–1632.

31 Meyer-Hoffert U, Wu Z, Schroder JM: Identification of lympho-epithelial Kazal-type inhibitor 2 in human skin as a kallikrein-related peptidase 5-specific protease inhibitor. PLoS One 2009;4:e4372.

32 Brattsand M, Stefansson K, Hubiche T, Nilsson SK, Egelrud T: SPINK9: a selective, skin-specific Kazal-type serine protease inhibitor. J Invest Dermatol 2009;129:1656–1665.

33 Roelandt T, Thys B, Heughebaert C, et al: LEKTI-1 in sickness and in health. Int J Cosmet Sci 2009;31:247–254.

34 Briot A, Deraison C, Lacroix M, et al: Kallikrein 5 induces atopic dermatitis-like lesions through PAR2-mediated thymic stromal lymphopoietin expression in Netherton syndrome. J Exp Med 2009;206:1135–1147.

35 Descargues P, Deraison C, Bonnart C, et al: Spink5-deficient mice mimic Netherton syndrome through degradation of desmoglein 1 by epidermal protease hyperactivity. Nat Genet 2005;37:56–65.

36 Fartasch M, Williams ML, Elias PM: Altered lamellar body secretion and stratum corneum membrane structure in Netherton syndrome: differentiation from other infantile erythrodermas and pathogenic implications. Arch Dermatol 1999;135:823–832.

37 Thorne EG, Zelickson AS, Mottaz JH, Katz HI, Deaton BH: Netherton's syndrome: an electronmicroscopic study. Arch Dermatol Res 1975;253:177–183.

38 Mevorah B, Frenk E: Ichthyosis linearis circumflexa Comel with trichorrhexis invaginata (Netherton's syndrome): a light-microscopic study of the skin changes. Dermatologica 1974;149:193–200.

39 Zina AM, Bundino S: Ichthyosis linearis circumflexa Comel and Netherton's syndrome: an ultrastructural study. Dermatologica 1979;158:404–412.

40 Frenk E, Mevorah B: Ichthyosis linearis circumflexa Comel with trichorrhexis invaginata (Netherton's syndrome): an ultrastructural study of the skin changes. Arch Dermatol Forsch 1972;245:42–49.

41 Hausser I, Anton-Lamprecht I, Hartschuh W, Petzoldt D: Netherton's syndrome: ultrastructure of the active lesion under retinoid therapy. Arch Dermatol Res 1989;281:165–172.

42 Nylander-Lundqvist E, Back O, Egelrud T: IL-1 beta activation in human epidermis. J Immunol 1996;157:1699–1704.

43 Elias PM: Stratum corneum architecture, metabolic activity and interactivity with subjacent cell layers. Exp Dermatol 1996;5:191–201.

44 Walley AJ, Chavanas S, Moffatt MF, et al: Gene polymorphism in Netherton and common atopic disease. Nat Genet 2001;29:175–178.

45 Al-Ghamdi F, Al-Raddadi A, Satti M: Peeling skin syndrome: 11 cases from Saudi Arabia. Ann Saudi Med 2006;26:352–357.

46 Janjua SA, Hussain I, Khachemoune A: Facial peeling skin syndrome: a case report and a brief review. Int J Dermatol 2007;46:287–289.
47 Hashimoto K, Hamzavi I, Tanaka K, Shwayder T: Acral peeling skin syndrome. J Am Acad Dermatol 2000;43:1112–1119.
48 Cassidy AJ, van Steensel MA, Steijlen PM, et al: A homozygous missense mutation in *TGM5* abolishes epidermal transglutaminase 5 activity and causes acral peeling skin syndrome. Am J Hum Genet 2005;77:909–917.
49 Kharfi M, El Fekih N, Ammar D, et al: A missense mutation in *TGM5* causes acral peeling skin syndrome in a Tunisian family. J Invest Dermatol 2009;129:2512–2515.
50 Candi E, Oddi S, Terrinoni A, et al: Transglutaminase 5 cross-links loricrin, involucrin, and small proline-rich proteins in vitro. J Biol Chem 2001;276:35014–35023.
51 Geyer AS, Ratajczak P, Pol-Rodriguez M, Millar WS, Garzon M, Richard G: Netherton syndrome with extensive skin peeling and failure to thrive due to a homozygous frameshift mutation in *SPINK5*. Dermatology 2005;210:308–314.
52 Komatsu N, Suga Y, Saijoh K, et al: Elevated human tissue kallikrein levels in the stratum corneum and serum of peeling skin syndrome-type B patients suggest an over-desquamation of corneocytes. J Invest Dermatol 2006;126:2338–2342.
53 Oji V, Eckl K, Aufenvenne K, et al: Loss of corneodesmosin leads to severe skin barrier defect, pruritus and atopy: unraveling the peeling skin disease. Am J Hum Genet 2010, in press.
54 Silverman AK, Ellis CN, Beals TF, Woo TY: Continual skin peeling syndrome: an electron microscopic study. Arch Dermatol 1986;122:71–75.
55 Brusasco A, Veraldi S, Tadini G, Caputo R: Localized peeling skin syndrome: case report with ultrastructural study. Br J Dermatol 1998;139:492–495.
56 Tsai K, Valente NY, Nico MM: Inflammatory peeling skin syndrome studied with electron microscopy. Pediatr Dermatol 2006;23:488–492.

Inherited Disorders of Corneocyte Proteins

4.1. The Keratinopathic Ichthyoses

4.1.1 Epidermolytic Ichthyosis (Epidermolytic Hyperkeratosis) and Superficial Epidermolytic Ichthyosis (Ichthyosis Bullosa of Siemens)

Clinical Characteristics

The newborn with epidermolytic ichthyosis (EI; OMIM No. 113800) typically presents with widespread areas of blistered or denuded skin. Because hyperkeratosis is usually not prominent, these newborns are initially often thought to have a form of epidermolysis bullosa or an autoimmune blistering disease. Only after the skin biopsy has demonstrated the characteristic histopathology of epidermolytic hyperkeratosis does the correct diagnosis become apparent. Morbidity and mortality are increased in these neonates because of widespread erosions that provide a portal for infection, and because of augmented fluid and electrolyte disturbances due to an abnormal barrier [1]. Because the fetus has a limited need for a competent permeability barrier in an aqueous, intrauterine environment, the mechanobullous phenotype predominates in newborns with EI (fig. 1). Yet, soon after birth (within weeks), the blistering tendency resolves and the phenotype shifts towards a hyperkeratotic/ichthyotic pattern. Thus, EI represents yet another example of an inherited skin disorder that displays a 'phenotypic shift' in response to movement from the hydrated in utero milieu to a desiccating external environment. This dramatic shift from a neonatal, mechanobullous to a postnatal hyperkeratotic phenotype is almost certainly driven by changes in environmental humidity (fig. 2).

Due to the blistering phenotype of the newborn, EI was previously termed 'bullous congenital ichthyosiform erythroderma' to distinguish it from the autosomal recessive, nonbullous group of autosomal recessive congenital ichthyoses (ARCI). Although the extent and severity of the mature phenotype vary greatly, it tends to remain similar within families [1]. At the severest end of the spectrum, EI involves the entire body surface with hyperkeratosis and scaling, accompanied by mechanical skin fragility (positive Nikolsky sign) and focal blistering, with an underlying erythroderma. However, not all patients with generalized involvement display an erythroderma, and many do not exhibit excessive skin fragility. When the palms and soles are spared, this feature usually indicates a keratin 10 (*K10;*

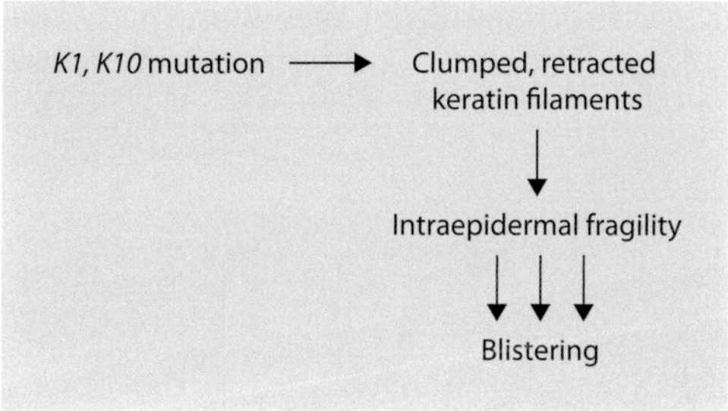

Fig. 1. Basis for pre- and perinatal phenotype of EI.

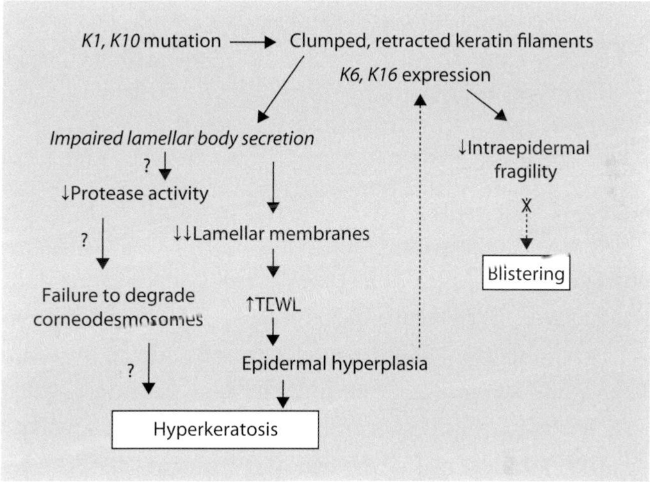

Fig. 2. Basis for postnatal phenotype of EI. TEWL = Transepidermal water loss.

OMIM No. 148080) rather than a *K1* (OMIM No. 139350) mutation; conversely, the palmar-plantar keratoderma can be quite severe in some *K1* mutations [2]. Typically, the hyperkeratosis in EI forms a ridged pattern, with accentuation of this feature in the flexures. However, scaling in some *K10* mutations can form an annular pattern [3–5]. Flexural scales often become secondarily colonized by bacteria, producing a foul odor. Finally, while the face is often involved, ectropion does not occur. In some EI patients, involvement may be more focal and limited to palms/soles, acral surfaces and/or the flexures. Variants with particularly widespread and thick, porcupine-like (hystrix-like) hyperkeratosis, which lack an earlier blistering phase, have been termed 'ichthyosis hystrix of Curth-Macklin' (OMIM No. 146600) [6].

Superficial EI (OMIM No. 600194), formerly called ichthyosis bullosa of Siemens, is a milder form of keratinopathic ichthyosis due to mutations in *K2*, a keratin that is transiently expressed in the stratum granulosum (SG). The superficial EI phenotype, though generalized, is milder than in EI, and blistering does usually not occur during

Table 1. Classification of keratinopathic ichthyoses

	Phenotype	Mutations
Autosomal dominant		
Epidermolytic ichthyosis[a]	classic	*K1*[b]*/K10*
Superficial epidermolytic ichthyosis[c]	less severe	*K2e*
Annular epidermolytic ichthyosis	annular	*K10*
Ichthyosis Curth-Macklin	hystrix-like	*K1*
Autosomal recessive		
Epidermolytic ichthyosis	severe classic	*K10*
Somatic		
Epidermolytic nevus	linear	*K1/K10* (mosaic)

[a] Also called epidermolytic hyperkeratosis, bullous ichthyosis, bullous ichthyosiform erythroderma.
[b] The *K1* variant is associated with palmar-plantar involvement and a milder phenotype.
[c] Also called ichthyosis bullosa of Siemens.

the perinatal period. However, because of a tendency for the stratum corneum (SC) to separate either at, or immediately below, the SG/SC interface, superficial EI often displays a peculiar type of superficial blistering or peeling termed the 'Maserung phenomenon' (resembling the texture of tree bark). The tendency for both EI and superficial EI to blister at the SG/SC interface can complicate therapy, because commonly deployed keratolytic agents and retinoids often remove too much SC, resulting in an eroded base (= 'therapeutic paradox') [7].

Biochemical Genetics

Keratins 1, 10 and 2 are expressed primarily, if not solely, in the epidermis, explaining the nonsyndromic nature of this group of disorders (table 1). The majority of mutations in *K1* (chromosome 12q13), *K2* (chromosome 12qB) and *K10* (chromosome 17q21–q22) are missense mutations [8–16], but in a significant minority of EI patients, no keratin mutations can be identified. Moreover, as many as 50% of all cases have no family history of disease, indicating a high frequency of spontaneous mutations. The majority of mutations involve highly conserved, helical boundary motifs [14, 17]. Although these keratinopathies are largely inherited as autosomal dominant traits, severe cases have been reported within consanguineous families with *K10* mutations (table 1) [18, 19]. These dominant-negative mutations result in expressed keratins that fail to form dimers, leading to disruption of intermediate filament formation (see below).

Localized forms of EI that are distributed along morphogenic lines (lines of Blaschko), i.e. epidermolytic epidermal nevi, are due to either chromosomal mosaicism or somatic (acquired) *K1* or *K10* mutations [5]. The offspring of patients with mosaic or nevoid variants of EI due to either *K1* or *K10* mutations are at risk for generalized forms of the disease [20].

Subcellular Pathogenesis

The main components of the intermediate filament network in the epidermis are the keratins, the most abundant proteins produced during the vectorial process of epidermal differentiation [21]. Typically, 1 acidic (type 1) keratin heterodimerizes with 1 basic (type 2) keratin, and 2 such dimers are arranged in an antiparallel and staggered configuration (protofilament) [22, 23]. In turn, 2 protofilaments comprise a protofibril, of which 4 protofibrils assemble to form a 10-nm-diameter intermediate filament. Within these filaments, the most abundant epidermal keratins, K1 and K10, eventually become linked to the cornified envelope [24–26].

K1 and *K10* mutations lead to dominant-negative 'clumping' of keratin pairs in suprabasal keratinocytes. Disruption of these filaments in turn results in retraction of intermediate filaments from beneath desmosomal plaques, forming clumps or perinuclear shells [27]. Underlying massive hyperkeratosis, a characteristic form of degeneration of the outer epidermal nucleated cell layers is observed, which stimulated the coinage of the term 'epidermolytic'. Basophilic intracellular deposits are present that resemble enlarged keratohyalin granules but instead are composed of clumped keratin filaments [28]. However, these changes may be focal or quite subtle in some patients: importantly, we have identified these changes ultrastructurally in several cases where the light-microscopic features were not diagnostic.

The need for a competent permeability barrier becomes paramount after birth, which stimulates homeostatic repair responses (initiated by loss of extracellular calcium and inflammatory cytokine activation), resulting in induction of epidermal hyperplasia (fig. 2). This response is paralleled by upregulation of the wound-healing keratins, K6 and K16 [29–31], and also activation of c-*myc* and 14-3-3 proteins [32]. Increased expression of K6 and K16 has been observed both in humans with EI [33, 34] and in mouse models [8, 35–37]. Thus, amelioration of the blistering phenotype in EI may be due to: (1) downregulation of mutant K1 and K10 under conditions of epidermal hyperplasia and/or (2) partial substitution of hyperproliferative K6/16 for K1/10, forming more functionally normal pairs of keratin filaments [35, 36, 38] (fig. 2).

The characteristic postnatal phenotype of EI is again 'driven' by a prominent permeability barrier abnormality [39]. Whereas basal transepidermal water loss (TEWL) rates are markedly elevated in most cases of EI (approx. threefold increase), barrier recovery kinetics are faster than in age-matched, control skin [40]. Both the cornified

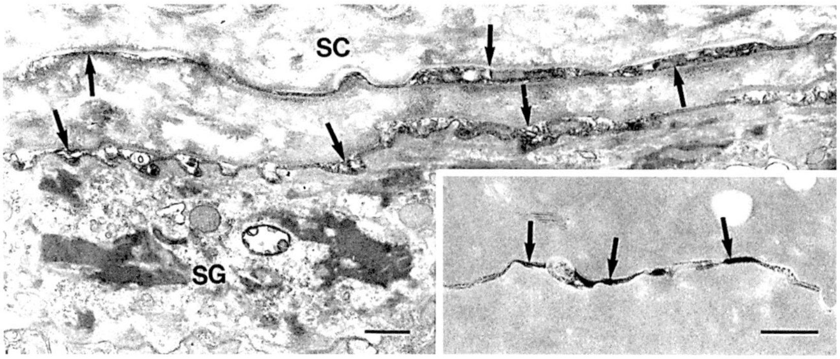

Fig. 3. Barrier dysfunction in EI. The lanthanum tracer (arrows) moves outward from the SG through the SC in a paracrine fashion (modified from Schmuth et al. [40]). Magnification bars = 0.5 μm.

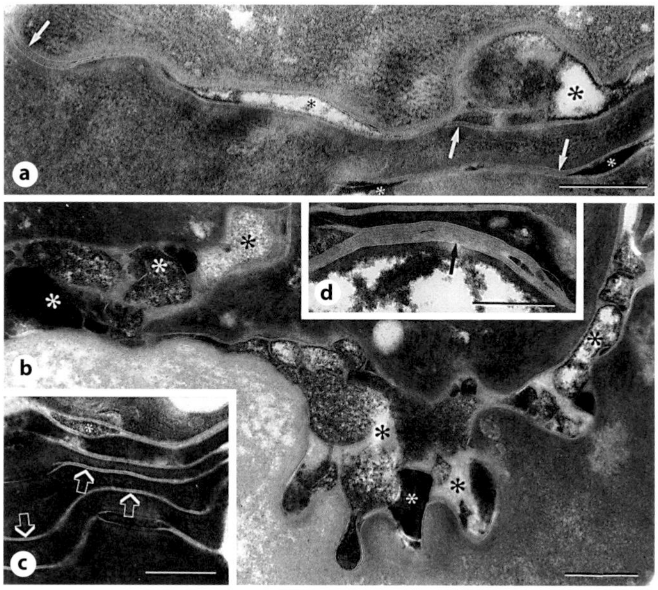

Fig. 4. Reduced extracellular lamellar bilayers (**a**, **c**, arrows) in EI, replaced with amorphous, nonlamellar material (**a**, **b**, asterisks). **d** Lamellar bilayers from a normal control (modified from Schmuth et al. [40]). Magnification bars = 0.5 μm.

envelope and the adjacent corneocyte lipid envelope are normal, eliminating a scaffold abnormality as an explanation for the barrier abnormality in EI. Although the increased fragility of the upper nucleated cell layers has been suggested to be the cause of the barrier abnormality [32], the water-soluble tracer colloidal lanthanum penetrates instead through the extracellular compartment, i.e. *between* and *not through* the cells [40]. Thus, despite the fragility of nucleated keratinocytes in EI, tracer permeates via the extracellular route (fig. 3).

The increased paracellular permeability in EI correlates with both decreased quantities and defective organization of extracellular lamellar bilayers, which are largely

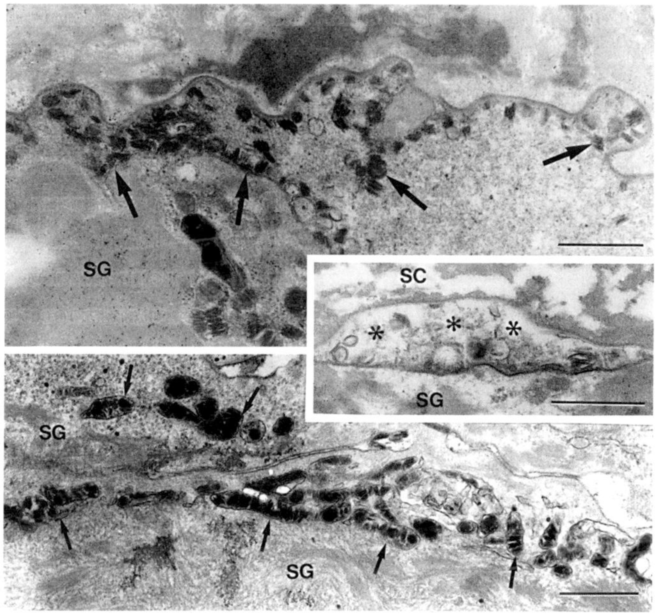

Fig. 5. Impaired secretion entombs lamellar bodies within corneocytes in EI (open arrows): amorphous extracellular material (asterisks) and reduced lamellar bilayers (modified from Schmuth et al. [40]). Magnification bars = 0.25 μm.

replaced by amorphous material [40] (fig. 4, 5). Both of these features, in turn, can be attributed to a blockade of secretion of lamellar body contents from granular cells, resulting in entombment of unsecreted lamellar bodies within corneocytes [40] (fig. 5, 6). The defect in secretion can be demonstrated independently by ultracytochemistry, which demonstrates little delivery of hydrolase activity to the extracellular spaces, with most lamellar body content markers instead becoming retained within corneocytes (fig. 7).

This secretory defect can be temporarily overridden, however, since acute barrier disruption induces a rapid release of preformed lamellar body contents, in conjunction with accelerated organelle secretion. Loss of calcium from the outermost granular layer perhaps provides the signal for the rapid exocytosis of lamellar bodies in conjunction with normalized repair kinetics [41], thereby accounting for the parallel acceleration of recovery kinetics in EI [40]. Thus, the baseline permeability barrier abnormality in EI can be attributed to impaired lamellar body secretion (resulting in deficiency of lamellar membranes), rather than to either corneocyte fragility or an abnormal cornified envelope scaffold (fig. 8). Our suggestion that impaired lamellar body secretion could reflect disruption of the cytoskeleton [40] is supported by similar observations in other secretory cells [42]. Whether the impaired desquamation in EI also results in a failure to deliver lamellar-body-derived desquamatory proteases still needs to be investigated (fig. 8). Likewise, the increased infection rates in EI could reflect a parallel failure to deliver lamellar-body-derived antimicrobial peptides (fig. 8), a feature that has not yet been

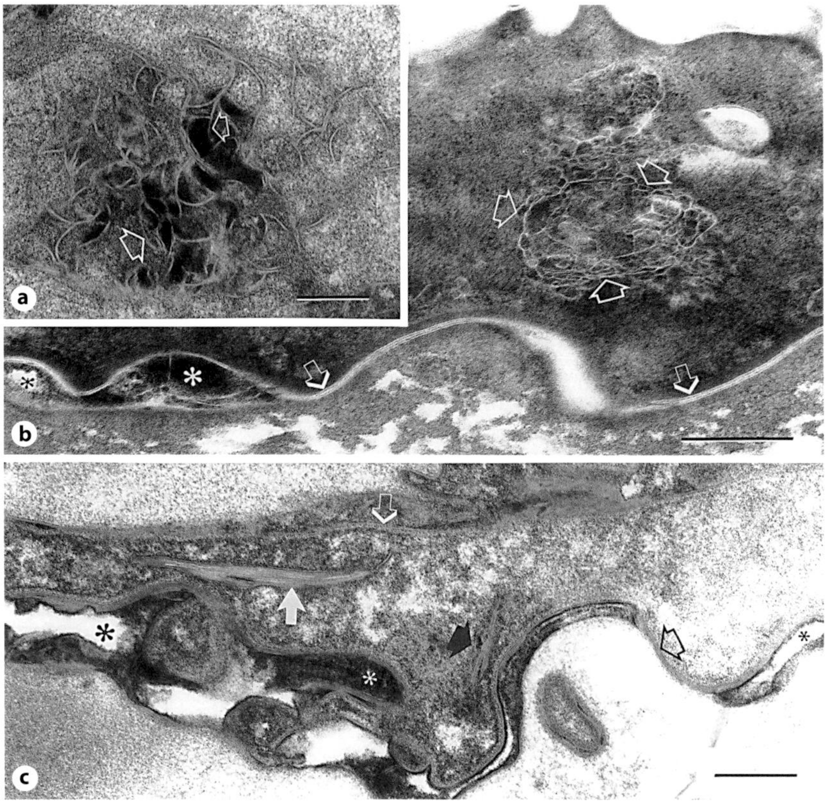

Fig. 6. Failure of lamellar body exocytosis in EI. Note arrays of unsecreted lamellar bodies in the peripheral cytosol of granular cells (SG; **a**, **b**, arrows). **c** Reduced secreted material at SG/SC interface; asterisks = spaces devoid of lamellar material (modified from Schmuth et al. [40]). Magnification bars = 0.5 µm.

assessed either. Nevertheless, these studies demonstrate that the intermediate filament framework plays a key role in regulating lamellar body secretion in normal keratinocytes.

Diagnostic Ultrastructure

In summary, both the cornified envelope and the corneocyte lipid envelope are normal in EI. Moreover, lamellar bodies are formed in normal numbers and exhibit normal lamellar contents. The key abnormalities are as follows. First, keratin filaments are clumped, often forming perinuclear shells, within granular and spinous cell layers. Second, rather than being secreted in toto at the SG/SC interface, lamellar bodies accumulate at the cell periphery, often forming long arrays just beneath the plasma membrane. Third, as a result of impaired secretion, many, if not most, lamellar bodies become entombed within corneocytes. Fourth, and finally, there is a paucity of lamellar bilayers in the SC extracellular spaces [40]. These ultrastructural features,

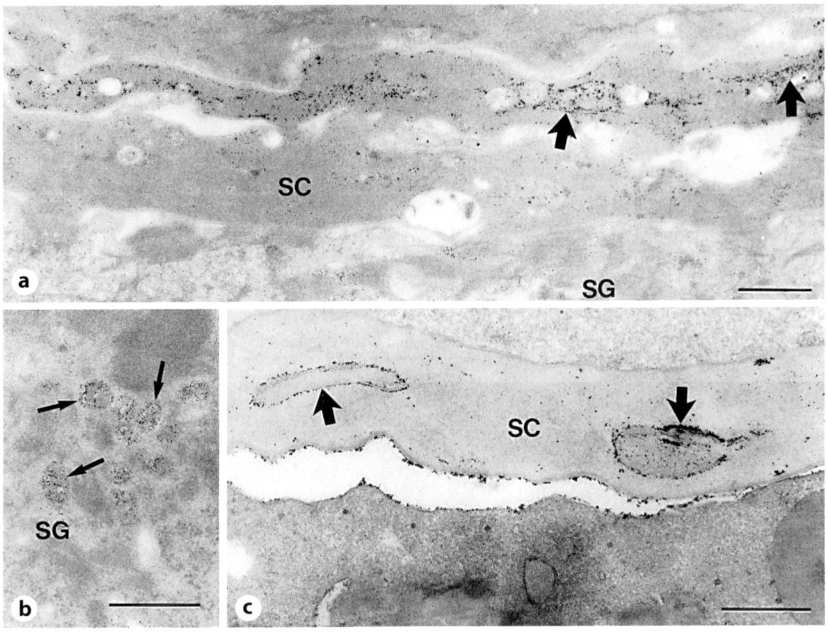

Fig. 7. Abnormal secretion demonstrated by ultrastructural cytochemistry in EI. Note the presence of substantial enzyme activity within corneocytes (**a**, **c**, arrows). In normal SC, all enzyme activity is restricted to the extracellular spaces (not shown) (modified from Schmuth et al. [40]). Magnification bars = 0.5 μm.

i.e. impaired secretion, coupled with a paucity of extracellular lamellar bilayers, along with clumping of keratin filaments within the granular and spinous cell layers, are diagnostic of EI.

4.2. Disorders of the Corneocyte Envelope

4.2.1 Autosomal Recessive Congenital Ichthyoses (TGM1 Mutations)

Clinical Characteristics

Of the many genes implicated in autosomal recessive congenital ichthyoses (ARCI), a variety of loss-of-function mutations in transglutaminase 1 (*TGM1*), which localizes to chromosome 14 [43–46], are most common, accounting for over a third of this group [47]. The most typical phenotype of TGM-1-linked ARCI is that of (classic) lamellar ichthyosis (LI; OMIM No. 1901995 and 242300), with large, dark, plate-like scales and variable underlying erythema [48]. The TGM-1-negative phenotype can also manifest as a finer, lighter scaling pattern, often with prominent erythema, i.e. a typical congenital ichthyosiform erythroderma phenotype, as well

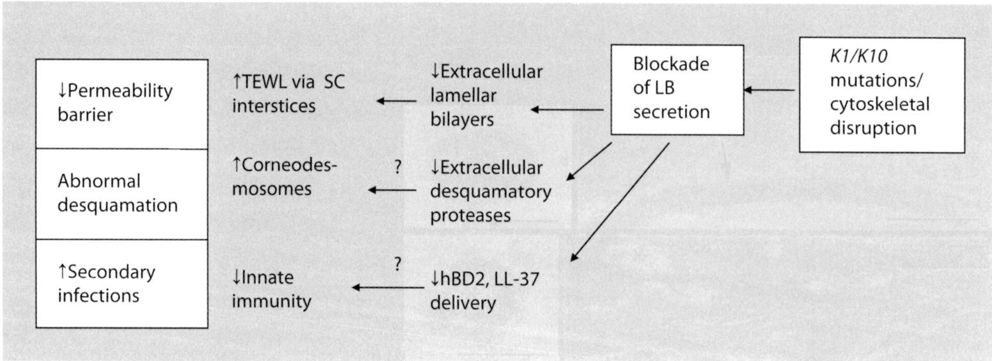

Fig. 8. Pathogenesis of EI. LB = Lamellar body.

as intermediate phenotypes [1]. Patients often display marked facial tautness with severe ectropion. Most if not all patients with *TGM1* mutations present at birth encased in a shiny, coherent 'collodion membrane'. As this hyperkeratotic membrane is shed during the first postnatal weeks, it is replaced by scaling and lichenification that involves the entire body surface, including the face and intertriginous areas, as well as the scalp, palms and soles. Yet, with few exceptions (see below), correlations between specific *TGM1* mutations and phenotypes within the ARCI spectrum have not emerged, in part because phenotypes are not stable over time and also in part because many patients are receiving drugs, such as retinoids, which modify the phenotype.

TGM1 mutations are also a cause of the 'self-resolving collodion baby' (OMIM No. 242300), in which the collodion membrane largely resolves into a very mild, generalized-scaling phenotype [49–51]. The phenomenon is not restricted to *TGM1* mutations; in fact, both nonsense and missense *ALOX* mutations (both *ALOX12B* and *ALOXE3*) are a more common cause of this phenotype in Scandinavians [51]. Certain *TGM1* mutations (p.Gly278Arg and p.Asp490Gly) in 'self-resolving collodion babies' may render the enzyme less active in a fully hydrated environment [52] (also cited in Akiyama [53]). Molecular modeling and enzyme assays suggest that the p-AspGly binds water, while the enzyme still resides in an inactive *trans*-conformation in utero, but after birth, with an increase in postnatal water loss, TGM-1 isomerizes back to a partially active *cis*-configuration [52].

Another *TGM1* variant, 'bathing suit ichthyosis' (OMIM No. 242300), denotes a phenotype in which pronounced scaling is restricted to a 'bathing suit' distribution and other flexures, sparing the face and extremities [54]. This phenotype has been attributed to *TGM1* mutations in which enzyme activity decreases at temperatures >33°C [55, 56]. Eight mutations in *TGM1* (Tyr276Asn, Arg126Cys, Arg264Trp, Arg307Gly, Arg264Gln, Arg687His, Arg315Cys and Arg315His) are associated with this variant and are proposed to alter the enzyme's hydrogen bonding [56].

Biochemical Genetics

Normally, the cornified envelope is assembled through TGM-1-mediated, calcium-dependent cross-linking of multiple peptide precursors via N-γ-glutamyl lysine isopeptide bonds. TGM-1 is a 92-kDa enzyme that is only expressed in the epidermis [57, 58]. Its predominant substrates are involucrin, loricrin and small proline-rich peptides [59]. Of these species, involucrin is incorporated first, with other peptides assembled beneath involucrin. Although other TGM types (i.e. TGM-3 and TGM-5) can also catalyze precursor cross-linking, the primary role of TGM-1 for this process is explained by its preferential tethering to the plasma membrane via myristate residues. It is this localization that places the enzyme in position to initiate cornified envelope formation [60]. Loss of TGM-1 function results in a defective cornified envelope at all levels of the SC [61, 62], a feature that distinguishes TGM-1-negative ARCI ultrastructurally from loricrin keratoderma (LK; see below). As noted above, a large proportion of the ARCI spectrum is caused by loss-of-function mutations in *TGM1*, with the net result being impaired cornified envelope structure and function [61]. To date, over 50 different *TGM1* mutations have been identified [61]. Ex vivo gene replacement of *TGM1*, followed by transplantation to SCID mice, successfully corrects the ARCI phenotype, including the barrier abnormality, in TGM-1-deficient ARCI [63].

Histopathology, Cellular Pathogenesis and Diagnostic Ultrastructure

The epidermis in TGM-1-deficient ARCI is acanthotic, often with a prominent granular layer. There is marked orthohyperkeratosis with occasional focal parakeratosis and a low-grade inflammatory infiltrate [48]. These histological features are consistent with a hyperplastic response to the barrier abnormality in LI, as occurs in the other diseases of cornification and as shown further in *Tgm1* knockout mice [64].

In TGM-1-negative ARCI, the resistance of corneocytes to boiling in sodium dodecyl sulfate and dithiothreitol is impaired due to attenuation of the corneocyte envelope, a potentially useful diagnostic feature [60, 65] (fig. 9). Moreover, despite clinically normal-appearing hair and nails, both of these tissues also are abnormally susceptible to detergent/dithiothreitol disruption, allowing provisional diagnosis without the need for skin biopsy [60, 66].

Ultrastructural studies reveal a range of abnormalities of the cornified envelope [61] (fig. 10). TGM-1-negative LI is associated with a prominent barrier abnormality [62]. Not only are basal TEWL levels elevated, but lanthanum tracer studies show that increased permeation is again *paracellular*; i.e. despite the defective corneocyte envelope, water permeates through the *extracellular* spaces [62] (fig. 11).

The basis for the barrier abnormality in TGM-1-negative ARCI is the fragmentation and truncation of the extracellular lamellar arrays [62] (fig. 12, 13). Minor abnormalities in the spacing of lamellar bilayers are also seen with RuO_4 postfixation for electron microscopy [67], and by X-ray diffraction [68], but it is doubtful that these minor changes account for the observed increase in rates of TEWL [62, 67–69]. Instead, increased movement of water between truncated membrane arrays appears

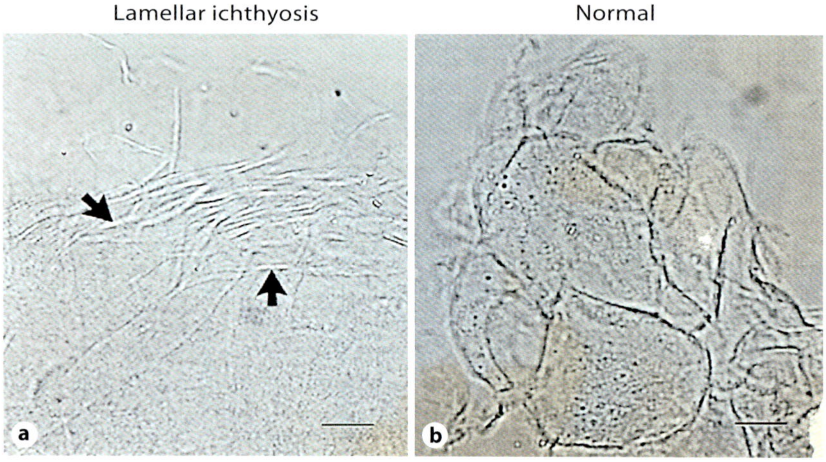

Fig. 9. Detergent and reducing agents disrupt TGM-1-negative ARCI scales (arrows) (modified from Rice et al. [60]). Magnification bars = 10 µm. **a** LI. **b** Normal.

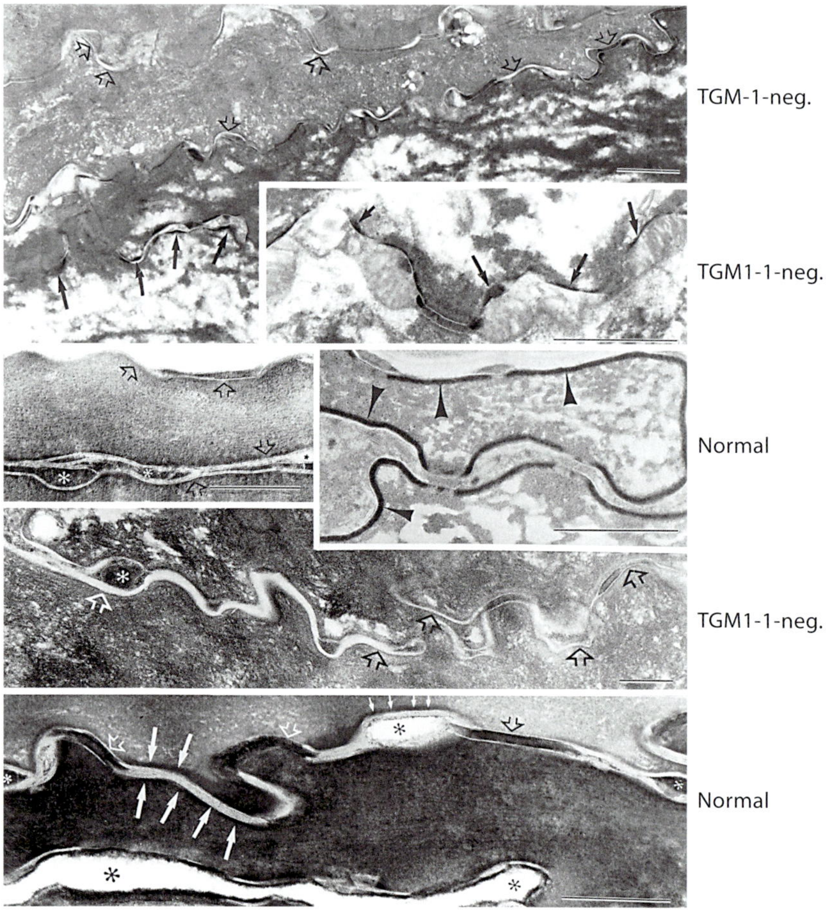

Fig. 10. Absent-to-attenuated cornified envelopes in TGM-1-negative ARCI (open arrows) (modified from Elias et al. [62]). Magnification bars = 0.25 µm.

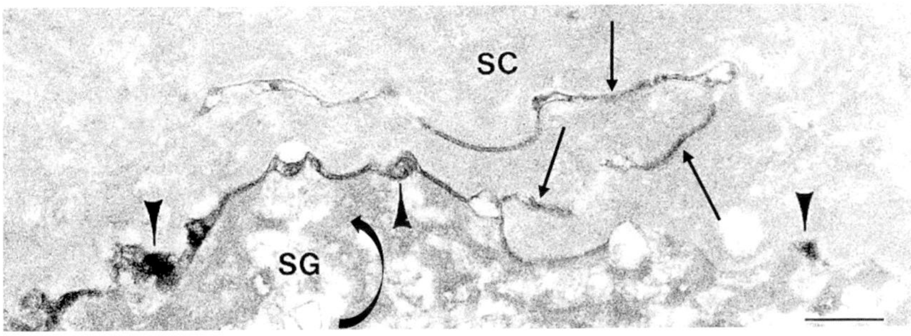

Fig. 11. Lanthanum perfusion demonstrates paracellular barrier abnormality in TGM-1-negative ARCI; the curved arrow indicates the direction of tracer perfusion; arrowheads indicate tracer in the extracellular compartment (modified from Elias et al. [62]). Magnification bar = 0.25 μm.

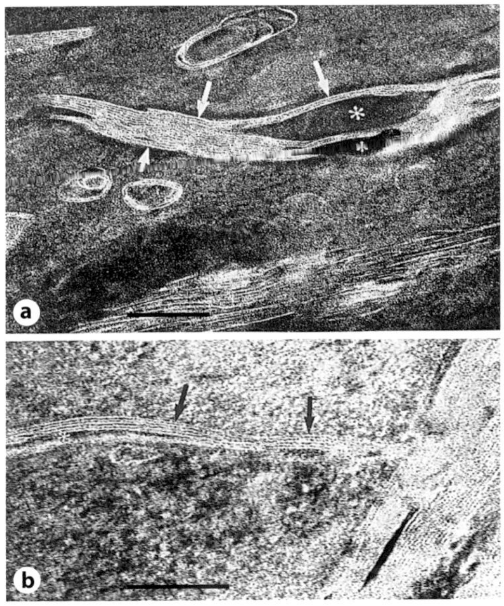

Fig. 12. Fragmentation of lamellar arrays adjacent to abnormal cornified envelopes in TGM-1-negative ARCI: prominent abnormalities in extracellular lamellar membranes are evident ultrastructurally (**a**), with truncation and fragmentation of extracellular lamellar membrane arrays in regions where the cornified envelope is attenuated (**a**, **b**, asterisks) (modified from Elias et al. [62]). Magnification bars = 0.1 μm.

to be the key determinant [62] (fig. 13). On electron microscopy of the SC, cornified envelopes are focally attenuated at all levels of the SC, while the corneocyte lipid envelope remains normal throughout [61, 62, 70]. This corneocyte abnormality is a diagnostic feature of TGM-1-negative ARCI, changes that otherwise are only seen in the *lower* SC of LK [71] (see below). Areas in which the extracellular lamellae are preserved correspond to regions in which the cornified envelope is present (shown schematically in fig. 13). Thus, the corneocyte envelope is required for the organization of lamellar arrays, which accounts for the barrier defect in TGM-1 deficiency [62], but TGM-1 is not involved in the formation of the corneocyte lipid envelope, since this

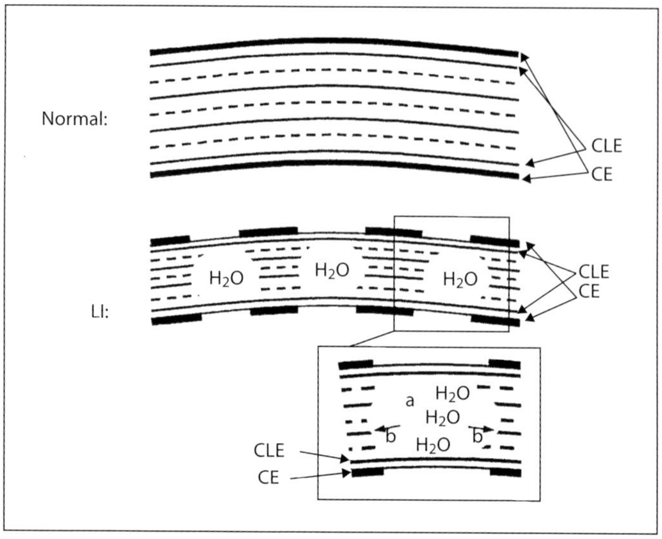

Fig. 13. Schematic basis for barrier abnormality in LI (modified from Elias et al. [62]).

structure is fully preserved. Therefore, enzyme(s) other than TGM-1 likely ω-esterify hydroxyceramides to the outer surface of the cornified envelope.

4.2.2 Loricrin Keratoderma

Clinical Characteristics

LK (OMIM No. 152445) exhibits a honeycomb-like palmar-plantar keratoderma as well as knuckle pads on the dorsum of the fingers, and often constricting bands encircling the fingers and/or toes (pseudoainhum), in association with generalized fine scaling [71–78]. This distinct phenotype is also referred to as Vohwinkel syndrome with ichthyosis, the Camisa variant of Vohwinkel syndrome or Vohwinkel disease limited to the skin. The features of the palmar-plantar keratoderma are similar to those of classic connexin-26-related Vohwinkel syndrome (OMIM No. 121011) [72], but LK lacks the neurosensory deafness of classic Vohwinkel syndrome, and Vohwinkel syndrome does not exhibit a generalized ichthyosis. Although the neonatal phenotype of LK is not well described, it can present with a collodion membrane phenotype [79]. The authors have observed 1 LK infant, who presented with exaggerated neonatal desquamation that evolved into a mild congenital ichthyosiform erythroderma phenotype. In some LK patients, the classic honeycombed pattern in the keratoderma is not evident, and the distal digits are tapered rather than constricted by keratotic bands, as occurs in Vohwinkel syndrome [1]. LK should be considered in any disorder of cornification patient with a mild, congenital ichthyosiform erythroderma phenotype in which palmar-plantar involvement is disproportionately severe.

Biochemical Genetics

LK is caused by dominantly inherited, frameshift mutations in the loricrin gene, which is localized within the epidermal differentiation complex on chromosome 1q21 [80]. Loricrin is a glycine-serine-cysteine-enriched protein, synthesized in the SG, that localizes either to distinct, L-type keratohyalin granules or at the periphery of filaggrin (FLG)-enriched keratohyalin granules [81–83]. Late in epidermal differentiation, loricrin migrates to the cell periphery, where it is deposited beneath involucrin residues, then becoming cross-linked to several other corneocyte envelope proteins (e.g. small proline-rich proteins, elafin, repetin, S100 proteins and approx. 20 other peptides) by TGM-1 to form the cornified envelope [59]. Normally, loricrin comprises up to 80% of the cornified envelope protein mass [59]. In LK, mutations result in elongation of the C-terminal domain of the loricrin protein, which misdirects the mutant peptide towards nuclei of the granular layer [84]. Thus, the mutant loricrin fails to reach the cornified envelope, but it instead remains tethered to the nucleus in the SG and parakeratotic SC [80, 84, 85]. The extent to which this aberrant nuclear localization modifies or impedes epidermal differentiation is unclear. Though cornified envelopes, deficient in loricrin, are thinner than in the normal SC [71], by the mid-to-outer SC, ongoing TGM-1-mediated cross-linking of other peptides [86] normalizes cornified envelope thickness [71].

Cellular Pathogenesis and Diagnostic Ultrastructure

In LK, the epidermis exhibits epidermal hyperplasia, hypergranulosis, marked hyperparakeratosis and parakeratosis, with characteristic round (rather than flattened) retained nuclei in the lower SC [75, 80]. As a result of attenuated cornified envelopes, granular layer and lower corneocyte integrity is impaired (fig. 14–16), but patients do not complain of increased blistering [71].

SC hydration is markedly decreased in hyperkeratotic/honeycomb-type skin sites. Basal TEWL rates are increased in non-palmar-plantar skin, and barrier recovery kinetics accelerate in comparison to normal skin [71]. The increased water loss, again, occurs predominantly via the paracellular route (fig. 15). The barrier abnormality can be attributed to disorganization of lamellar bilayers adjacent to areas of attenuated cornified envelope, and, as in TGM-1-negative LI, the water-soluble, electron-dense tracer lanthanum penetrates through these disorganized extracellular domains (fig. 15 and 17). In contrast to TGM-1-deficient ARCI, cornified envelopes in LK are attenuated only in the lower SC, and their dimensions normalize in the outer SC (fig. 16b), likely due to ongoing compensatory incorporation of other cornified envelope precursor peptides (fig. 16b, 17).

This normalization of cornified envelope dimensions in the mid-to-outer SC correlates with the presence of abundant calcium in the SC extracellular spaces (due to the defective barrier), where it is correctly positioned to activate TGM-1 and allow ongoing enzyme activity [71]. As in TGM-1-negative ARCI, lamellar bilayer abnormalities occur adjacent to regions in which discontinuities and attenuation of the

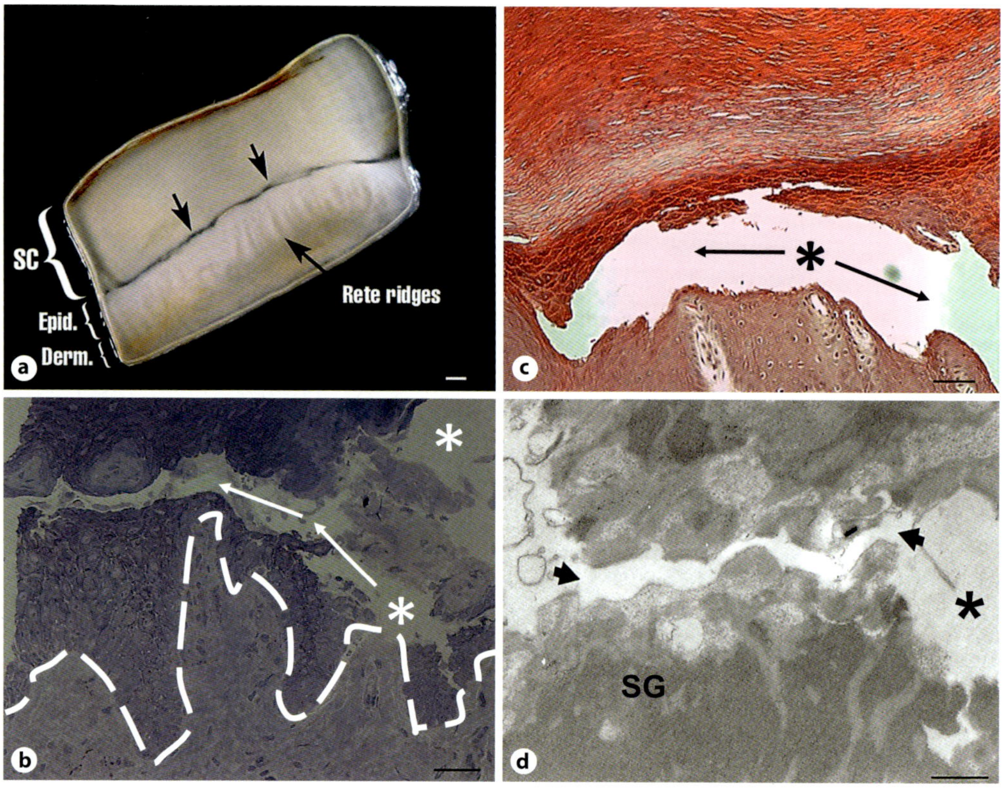

Fig. 14. Skin fragility localizes to the outer granular layer. Cleavage plane in mechanically induced fracture of patient samples passes both between and across cells of the outer granular layer (SG); asterisks = clefts; arrows = direction of cleavage plane (modified from Schmuth et al. [71]). **a** Dark-field view of thick section. Magnification bar = 1 µm. **b** Hematoxylin and eosin. Magnification bar = 10 µm. **c** Toluidine-blue-stained semithin preparation. Magnification bar = 10 µm. **d** OsO_4-postfixed ultrathin section at the level of the outer SG. Magnification bar = 0.5 µm.

cornified envelope are present, but in LK, these sites are largely restricted to the lower SC (fig. 17). The primary pathogenic role of the scaffold abnormality is underscored by the presence of a normal lamellar body secretory system, with largely unimpeded secretion of lamellar body contents, a normal corneocyte lipid envelope and normal bound ω-hydroxyceramide content [71].

In summary, the permeability barrier abnormality in LK can be attributed to a defective cornified envelope scaffold in the lower SC layers (fig. 18). The ultrastructural diagnosis can be made by comparing cornified envelope structure and dimensions in the lower versus outer SC, and identification of a cleavage plane in the outermost SG and lower SC. Thus, both TGM-1-deficient ARCI and LK share a common disease pathomechanism. In TGM-1-deficient ARCI, the enzyme responsible for cross-linking protein is defective, while in LK, its major substrate is deficient (fig. 18).

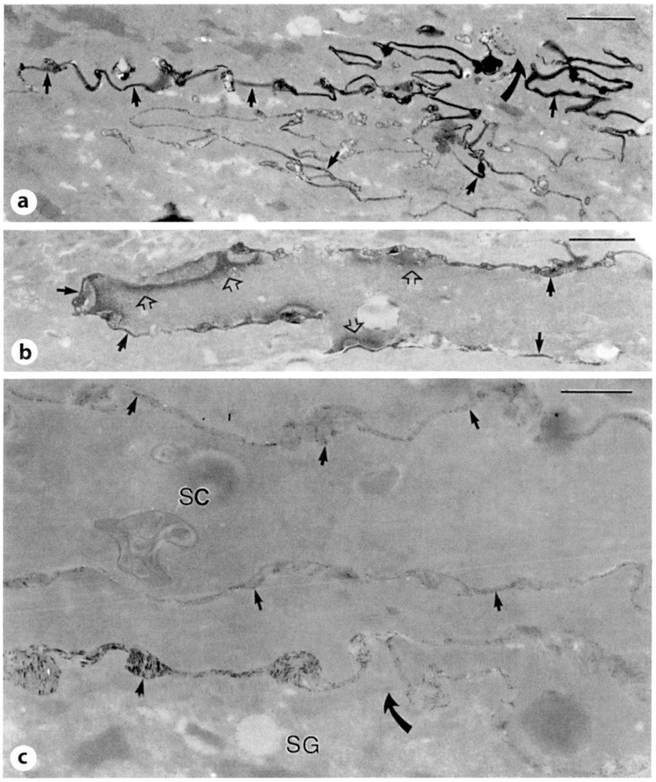

Fig. 15. Increased permeability occurs primarily via the extracellular pathway in LK. Despite evidence of keratinocyte fragility, water-soluble, electron-dense tracer (colloidal lanthanum) largely traverses the SC via extracellular domains (arrows). Some corneocytes in the lower SC demonstrate (curved arrows) evidence of fragility, shown by leakage of tracer into the cytosol (**b**, open arrows) (modified from Schmuth et al. [71]). **a**, **b** OsO_4 postfixation. **a**, **b** Magnification bars = 1 µm. **c** Magnification bar = 0.5 µm.

4.2.3 Ichthyosis Vulgaris

Clinical Characteristics

Ichthyosis vulgaris (IV; OMIM No. 146700) represents the most common disorder of cornification. Estimates of its prevalence range widely, undoubtedly because it is often difficult to distinguish between IV and xerosis, particularly the dry skin of atopic dermatitis (AD), which is a manifestation of the same genetic trait (i.e. *FLG* mutations). Thus, previously reported prevalence data, ranging from 1 in 250 in British schoolchildren [87] to studies from Japan [88] and Mexico [89], which estimated substantially lower prevalences (i.e. 1:1,000–2,000), are likely underestimates.

While a phenotype is rarely present in neonates with IV, the disease usually becomes evident by 3 months of age and is characterized by rather mild, generalized fine scaling with sparing of the face and flexures. The extensor surfaces of the extremities are more affected than is the trunk. Involvement of the palms and soles (hyperlinearity) is typical. Keratosis pilaris and AD are present in most patients. It is difficult, if not impossible, to differentiate clinically between the phenotype of IV and the xerosis that accompanies AD. Indeed, recent studies in FLG-deficient mice suggest that they are one and the same, and reflect, in part, low-grade inflammation [90, 91].

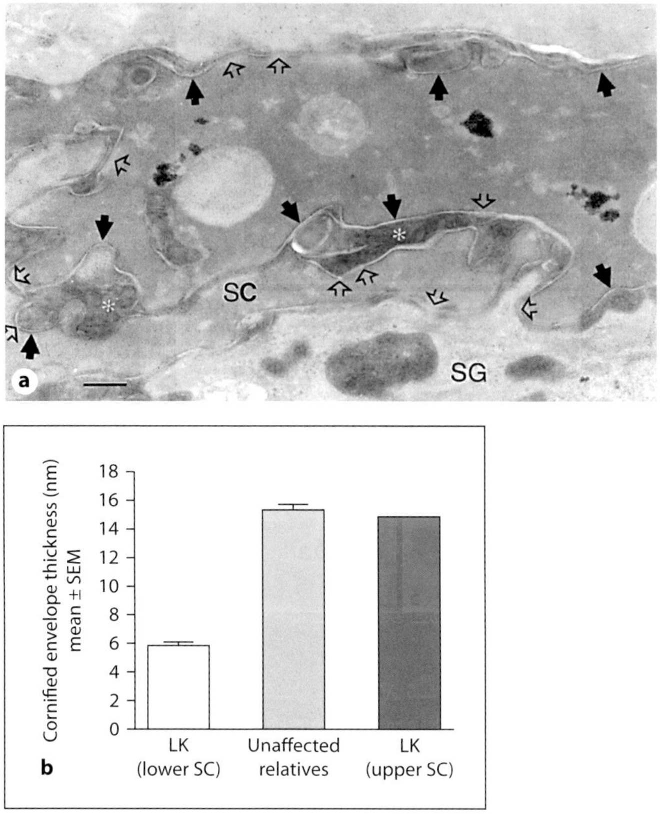

Fig. 16. Cornified envelopes are attenuated only in the lower SC in LK. **a** Note cornified envelopes with frequent discontinuities (open arrows) in the lower SC in LK versus those with normal dimensions in control and upper SC of LK (modified from Schmuth et al. [71]). Magnification bar = 0.25 μm.

IV is a semidominant trait, exhibiting a severer phenotype when both alleles are affected. Heterozygous patients generally display a mild or minimal 'xerotic' phenotype, while homozygous and compound heterozygous *FLG* genotypes exhibit the full IV phenotype [92]. The high overall prevalence of *FLG* mutations in the population, even in phenotypically normal subjects, suggests that FLG deficiency may confer some as yet unknown, evolutionary advantage(s). As noted above, the same *FLG* mutations have been linked to AD [93, 94], and AD frequently overlaps with IV, raising questions about the potential role of additional exogenous stressors in provoking a phenotypic shift from IV to AD [95, 96].

Biochemical Genetics

Mutations in the gene (*FLG*) that encodes FLG, located in the epidermal differentiation complex on chromosome 1q21 [97, 98], cause IV [92–94, 99–101] (fig. 19). Up to 20 mutations have been described, with different spectra of alterations and prevalences in Northern Europeans, Austrians, Chinese and Japanese populations [for a review, see 1].

A primary abnormality in FLG has long been suspected to be the cause of IV, because pro-FLG and its dephosphorylated, proteolytic product FLG are reduced or

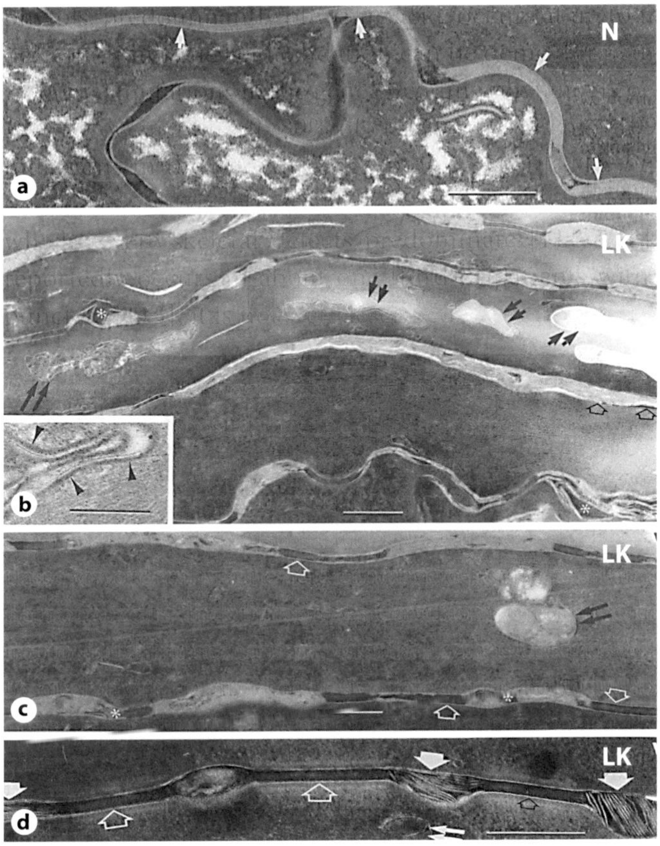

Fig. 17. Normal quantities but abnormal organization of extracellular lamellae in LK (modified from Schmuth et al. [71]). RuO_4 postfixation. Magnification bars = 0.25 µm. **a** Normal SC, extracellular lamellar bilayers (solid arrows). **b, c** Attenuated cornified envelopes are again evident throughout the lower SC. Although extensive extracellular arrays are present in LK, these bilayers are loosely organized and often fragmented in comparison to normal SC. Findings are comparable, but more exaggerated in severely (**b**) versus less severely involved (**c**) skin sites. **b, inset** Note cornified envelope of near-normal thickness in the outer SC of LK. Delayed lipid processing (**d**, solid arrows) can also be seen, and some entombed lamellar bodies are evident (**b–d**, double arrows). In contrast, the corneocyte lipid envelope is normal regardless of disease severity (**c**, **d**, open arrows).

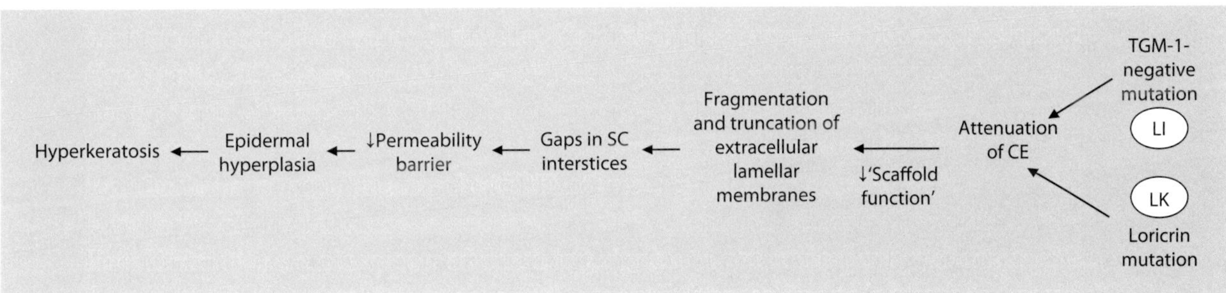

Fig. 18. Related pathogenesis of LK and TGM-1-negative ARCI. CE = Cornified envelope.

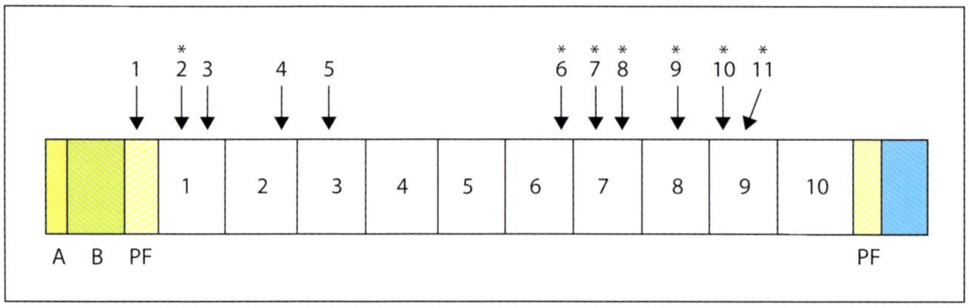

Fig. 19. Structure of human pro-FLG and mutations in IV: location of prevalent mutations is shown that are associated with IV and AD. The figure shows a pro-FLG molecule with 10 FLG repeats; the number of repeats can vary from 10 to 12. The mutations that are starred represent nonsense mutations; the remainder represent either insertion or deletion mutations, which all result in premature termination. The mutations shown are: 1 = 1249insG; 2 = Arg501stop; 3 = 2282del4; 4 = 3321delA; 5 = 3702delG; 6 = Glu2422stop; 7 = Arg2447stop; 8 = Ser2554stop; 9 = Ser2889stop; 10 = Ser3247stop; 11 = Ser3296stop. PF domains indicate the partial (half) FLG domains located at each end of FLG (modified from Presland [102]).

absent [103], correlating with a long-recognized paucity in F-type keratohyalin granules within the SG [104–106]. The delay in identifying the genetic basis of IV was due to the exceptionally long and highly repetitive sequence of the *FLG* gene. Many of the common mutations result in a decrease in the number of FLG repeats [102]. Interestingly, even in the absence of overt mutations, the number of repeats within the *FLG* gene varies from 10 to 12, which may account for subtle phenotypic variability in IV [107] and could help to explain certain discrepancies in prevalence data (see above).

However, some patients who bear certain distal mutations that impede processing of pro-FLG to FLG, may also accumulate pro-FLG, with reduced FLG [93]. Moreover, mice with deficiency of the pro-flg processing enzyme, matriptase (ST14), exhibit an ichthyotic phenotype (fig. 20) [108]; deficiency of ST14 is associated with a rare, recessive ichthyosiform dermatosis, associated with hypotrichosis (ARIH: OMIM 610765) [for classification, see chapter 1, this vol., pp. 1–29]). Likewise, mutant (flaky tail) mice, which bear a distal mutation in *Proflg* that blocks the conversion of pro-flg to flg [109], display a subtle barrier abnormality and decreased thresholds to the development of an AD-like dermatosis following exposure to haptens or allergens [90, 91]. These studies suggest that FLG deficiency alone, by provoking a barrier abnormality (see below), predisposes to the development of AD against a background of prior IV.

Cellular Pathogenesis

A histological feature of IV is a reduced or absent granular layer with a paucity of F-type keratohyalin granules and often reduced pro-FLG content [103, 106]. Pro-FLG is the initial translation product of the *FLG* gene. It is found in F-type

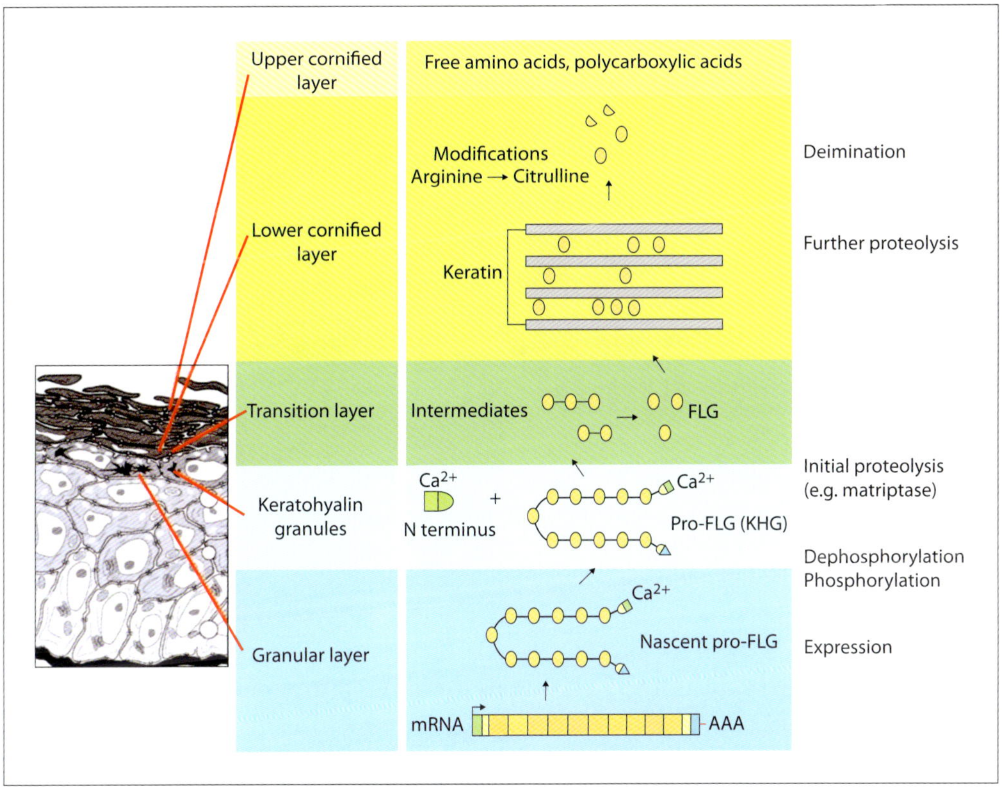

Fig. 20. Processing of pro-FLG during terminal differentiation. Pro-FLG is synthesized and phosphorylated in the granular layer and stored in keratohyalin granules (KHG). At the granular to cornified cell transition, pro-FLG is dephosphorylated and cleaved by proteases to FLG. The N terminus is cleaved from pro-FLG and associates with other proteins in the cytoplasm and nucleus. FLG aggregates keratin filaments in cornified cells (macrofibrils) that are retained in cornified cells. FLG is then graded by proteases. The resulting free amino acids and their deiminated products carry out various functions in the cornified cells (modified from Presland [102]). AAA = amino acid terminus.

keratohyalin granules in the granular layer of the epidermis, which is identified by this feature. Absence of the granular layer is independent of body site and season of the year but correlates with disease severity and mutational status [103, 106, 110–112]. Patients with 1 mutation (heterozygous) display a reduced granular layer, while patients with 2 *FLG* mutations (homozygotes or compound heterozygotes) usually lack a granular layer [99–101]. However, in rare cases, even patients with both alleles mutated can still show residual keratohyalin granules [113]. The persistence of F-type keratohyalin in some double-allele IV subjects appears to depend on the location of the mutation within the gene, i.e. more proximal mutations show complete absence of pro-FLG [114], while more distal mutations show residual, yet greatly reduced, truncated pro-FLG species that are not processed to FLG monomers [93].

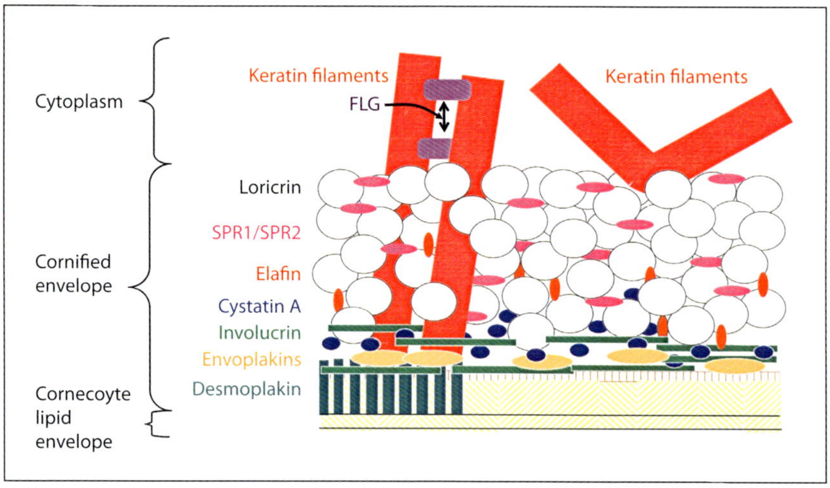

Fig. 21. Proposed localization of FLG within the cornified envelope (modified from Steinert and Marekov [59]). SPR = Small proline-rich protein.

Pro-FLG is a large, histidine-rich, highly cationic phosphoprotein, consisting of several FLG repeats, connected by peptide segments enriched in hydrophobic amino acids [82, 115]. During cornification, pro-FLG is dephosphorylated, proteolytically processed by matriptase into C-terminal FLG monomers (ST14), which then insert into the cornified envelope [116] (fig. 20 and 21). In contrast to the cytoplasmic location of the C-terminal FLG monomers, the N-terminal portion of pro-FLG is tethered to the nucleus, consistent with its nuclear localization sequence (S100-like EF hand domain). It has been proposed that this sequence may impart calcium-dependent, nuclear functions [117]. Later processing results in detachment of the C-terminal peptides that are further proteolyzed and deiminated into small, osmotically active, acidic molecules ('natural moisturizing factor').

Although FLG monomers are widely believed to mediate the collapse of the keratin filament network during cornification, keratin intermediate filament organization appears normal in the corneocyte cytosol of IV [103, 118], suggesting that FLG may not be required (or only a small amount of FLG is needed) for normal keratin aggregation. Pro-FLG is proteolyzed above the stratum compactum by arginine depeptidase and subsequently proteolyzed further into its constituent amino acids by an as yet uncharacterized protease (potentially the aspartate protease cathepsin D) [119], and finally deiminated into polycarboxylic acids [109, 120, 121]. These small acidic molecules include *trans*-urocanic acid and pyrrolidone carboxylic acid, which mediate much of the hygroscopic properties that underlie SC hydration [122]. In IV, affected corneocytes display a reduced capacity to imbibe water when exposed to a high humidity or during bathing, which could impair desquamation, since outer corneocytes cannot 'swell and slough' with bathing [123]. Thus, the scaling abnormality may be directly related

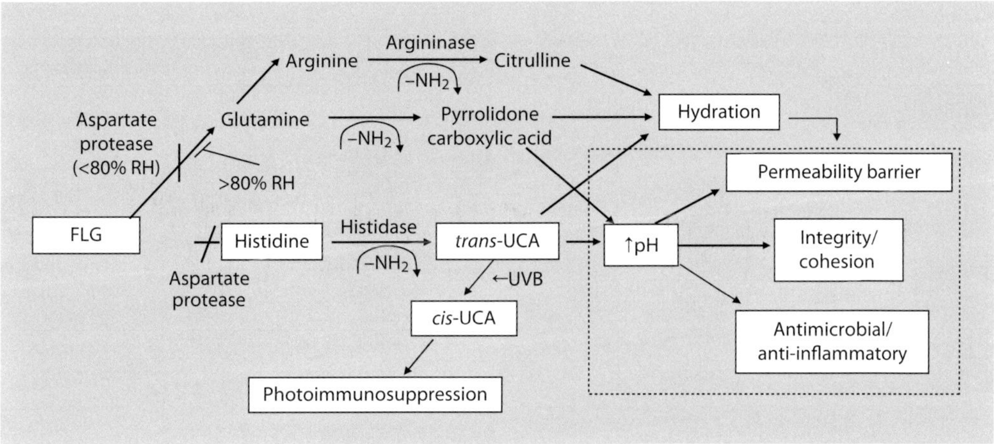

Fig. 22. The FLG proteolytic pathway impacts multiple SC functions in a pH-dependent fashion (modified from Elias et al. [95]). RH = Relative humidity; UCA = urocanic acid; UVB = ultraviolet B.

to the reduction in proteolytic breakdown products of FLG, resulting in a paucity of the osmotically active metabolites that regulate corneocyte hydration [120, 124, 125]. FLG hydrolysis accelerates with xeric stress (as relative humidity declines below 80%) [122]; the inability to accommodate to xeric stress by increased FLG hydrolysis could explain the exacerbation of xerosis during sustained exposure to a dry environment in IV. FLG deficiency in IV may also reduce SC acidification [126], thereby impairing several other critical SC functions (barrier function, SC cohesion and antimicrobial defense) by pH-related mechanisms [114] (fig. 22; see below).

Basis for the Barrier Abnormality in Ichthyosis Vulgaris

On electron microscopy, residual F-type keratohyalin granules have been described as being poorly formed ('crumbly') [127] or absent [106]. Preliminary studies in genotyped IV subjects and in FLG-deficient mouse models [90, 91] suggest that the phenotype in IV is linked, once again, to an underlying abnormality in permeability barrier homeostasis [128]. The pH of SC is elevated in IV [128, 129], and the increase in pH, in turn, could activate serine proteases (kallikreins), with a host of negative downstream consequences, including: (a) proteinase-activated-receptor-2-mediated blockade of lamellar body secretion [130, 131]; (b) possible downstream alterations in keratin filament organization that could impede lamellar body secretion (see below), and (c) both Th1- and kallikrein-5-activated Th2 inflammation [132] (fig. 23). According to this view, while the primary phenotype in IV is one of scaling, it also represents the *forme fruste* of AD, displaying clinical inflammation only when affected skin is either exposed to sustained antigen ingress and/or to additional acquired stressors to the barrier (e.g. high pH surfactants, exposure to a reduced external humidity or sustained psychological stress).

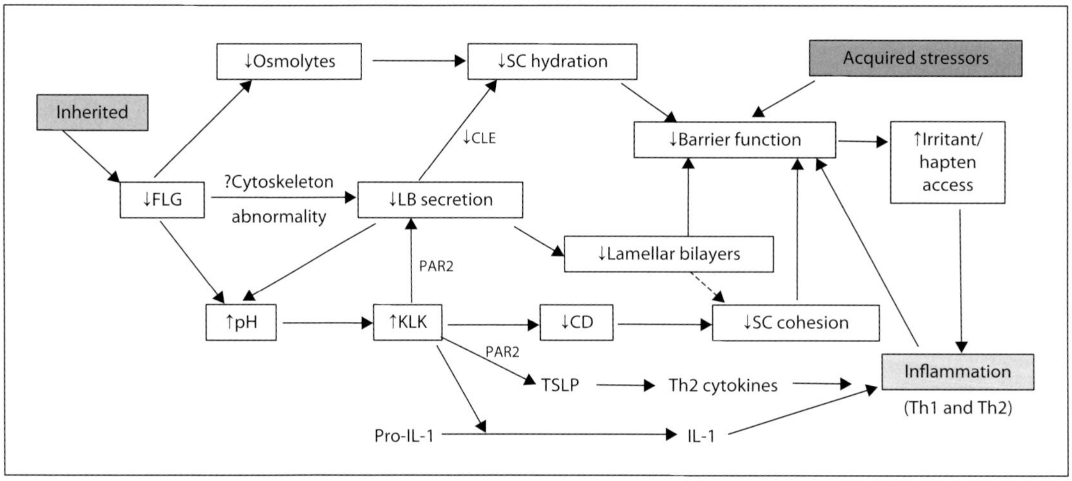

Fig. 23. Mechanisms whereby FLG deficiency in IV could predispose to the development of AD: decreased FLG leads to decreased levels of osmolytes, which in turn raise the pH of the SC. Decreased lamellar body (LB) secretion leads to decreased lamellar bilayers *and* a defective corneocyte lipid envelope (CLE), accounting in part for poor SC hydration. PAR2 = Proteinase-activated receptor 2; KLK = kallikrein; CD = corneodesmosomes; TSLP = thymocyte-stimulating lymphopoietin.

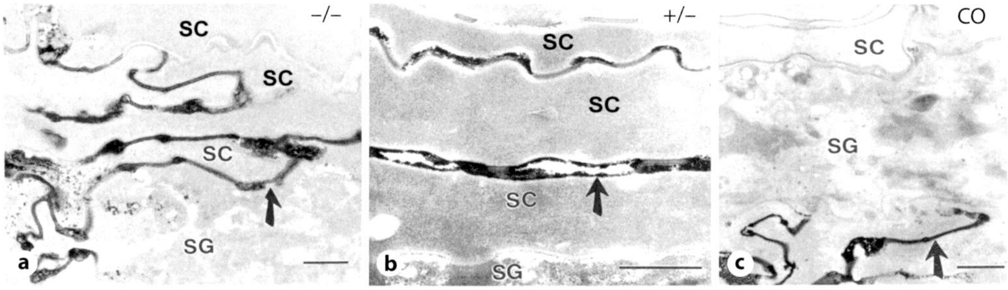

Fig. 24. Increased permeability of the SC occurs via the paracellular route in IV. Lanthanum tracer: –/– = patients with absent granular layer, with double-allele mutations; +/– = partial (reduced) granular layer; CO = age-matched normal control. Magnification bars = 0.5 μm.

Cellular Pathogenesis and Diagnostic Ultrastructure

Ultrastructural analysis is more sensitive in revealing a paucity/absence of F-type keratohyalin granules than either light microscopy or immunohistochemical visualization of epidermal FLG content [127]. Residual F-type keratohyalin exhibits a crumbly appearance in heterozygous individuals [133]. Both single- and double-allele IV exhibits an increased number of SC layers, which are nonetheless abnormally permeable to lanthanum tracer, indicative of barrier abnormality in both IV patients [128] and in mutant murine strains with reduced FLG [91]. As in all the other ichthyoses studied to date, increased permeation occurs via the extracellular route (fig. 24), i.e.

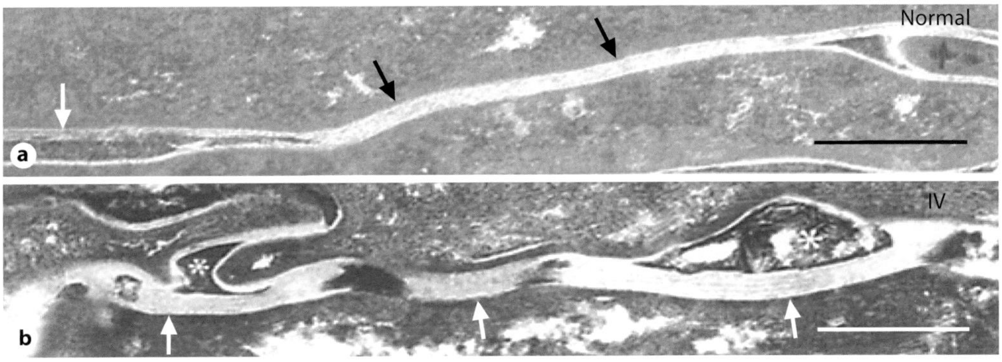

Fig. 25. Decreased number and abnormal organization of extracellular lamellar bilayers in IV. Magnification bars = 0.2 µm. **b** Reduced lamellar bilayers (arrows), and foci of intact lamellar bilayers are replaced/displaced by nonlamellar, amorphous material (asterisks) in a patient with double-allele *FLG* mutations. **a** Age-matched normal (control) SC.

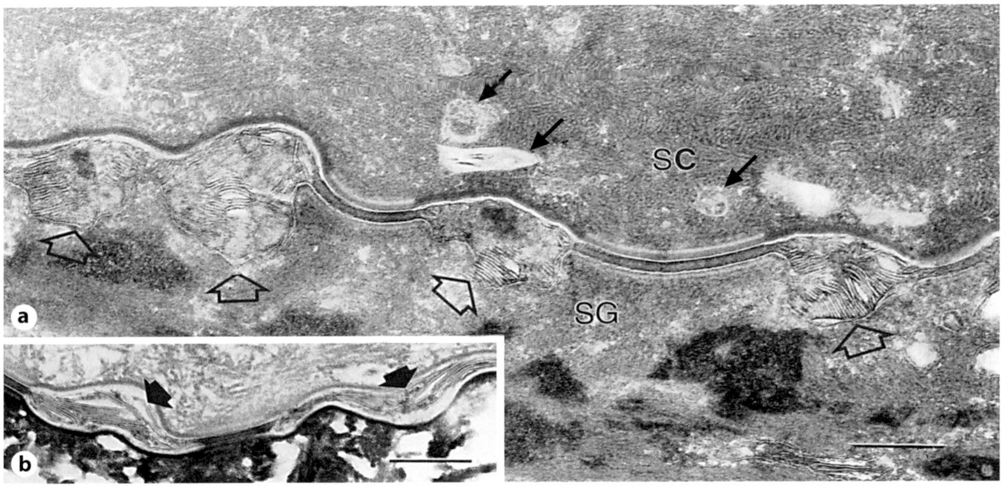

Fig. 26. Delayed maturation of lamellar bilayers in IV. Magnification bars = 0.2 µm. **a** Lamellar body formation is normal (open arrows), but secretion is incomplete (solid arrows). **b** 'Immature' bilayers persist within SC interstices (arrows), but corneodesmosomes and cornified envelopes appear normal.

despite abnormalities in corneocyte structural proteins, there is no evidence for transcellular permeability.

Furthermore, a partial impairment of lamellar body secretion results in both reduced numbers of extracellular lamellar bilayers (fig. 25b, open arrows) and displacement of bilayers by amorphous material (fig. 25b, asterisks).

Incompletely processed (immature) lamellar material persists several cell layers above the SG/SC junction (fig. 26). The lipid processing abnormality in IV likely results from an inverse relationship between residual levels of FLG expression and skin surface pH, i.e. homozygote IV patients with a complete lack of FLG display the highest skin surface pH [114] (fig. 23). The paucity of FLG and its downstream acidic, proteolytic products result in decreased activities of the 2 key ceramide-generating enzymes (β-glucocerebrosidase and acid sphingomyelinase), which display acidic pH optima. Although FLG is a component of the cornified envelope [116], it displays a largely normal structure and integrity in IV [Gruber, unpubl. data] (fig. 26). However, the corneocyte lipid envelope could repeatedly be functionally abnormal, because bound ω-OH ceramide levels are reduced [134]. However, a more systematic evaluation of corneocyte lipid envelope structure, composition and function would clearly be of interest.

Hence, despite FLG deficiency, there is no evidence of a scaffold abnormality in IV, as occurs in TGM-1-negative ARCI and LK. Instead, FLG-deficient IV shows the following ultrastructural abnormalities: (1) a reduced number of F-type keratohyalin granules; (2) impaired lamellar body secretion; (3) reduced extracellular lamellar bilayers, and (4) delayed maturation of lamellar membrane structures.

4.3. Ichthyosis en Confettis

4.3.1 Clinical Features

The phenotype of ichthyosis en confettis (IEC, congenital reticular ichthyosiform erythroderma, ichthyosis variegata) begins with generalized scaling, with a variable, but often intense, underlying erythroderma at or shortly after birth [135]. Although most cases reportedly represent single affected cases within kindreds, one of the authors (M.L.W.) has observed a mother with IEC who had 2 affected sons by different fathers, arguing strongly for a dominant inheritance pattern. While the range of severity among patients suggests that IEC could be genetically heterogeneous [135], some similar ultrastructural features have been found in several of our cases (n = 7; see below), suggesting instead mutations in a single or related group of gene(s) in all patients. In a very recent report, Choate et al. [136] demonstrated that several patients, inlucluding several of ours, display frameshift mutations in K10. The hallmark of IEC is the progressive appearance and enlargement of hundreds-to-thousands of white, confetti-like, nonscaling macules beginning in early childhood [135, 137, 138]. Choate et al. showed further that these white lesions are enriched with clones of keratinocytes in which the K10 mutations have reverted to normal [136]. Typically, these children are initially diagnosed with congenital ichthyosiform erythroderma, but after they begin to develop areas of macular leukoderma, the diagnosis of IEC becomes evident. Erythrodermic patients often display growth failure, due at least in part to a severe permeability barrier abnormality [139], while others display a milder, albeit generalized phenotype. Squamous cell carcinomas have been reported in these severely affected adults [140, 141]. Finally, some IEC patients exhibit a severe,

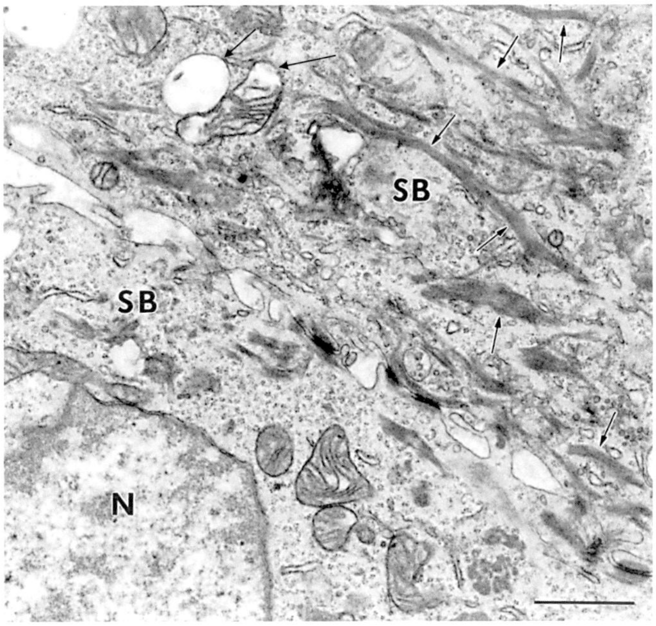

Fig. 27. Near-normal basal cells in involved skin of IEC. Note normal intermediate filament bundles in cytosol (arrows), but decreased/smaller desmosomes and early mitochondrial abnormalities can already be seen (arrows). N = Nucleus; SB = basal layer. Magnification bar = 1.0 µm.

erythrodermic phenotype, with islands of leukoderma, hair loss and underdeveloped ears, the so-called MAUIE syndrome for micropinnae, alopecia universalis, congenital ichthyosis and ectropion [140, 141].

4.3.2 *Pathology and Diagnostic Ultrastructure*

While the histology of white lesions appears normal, erythematous areas display acanthosis with hyperkeratosis, and flattening of the rete ridges [140]. The granular layer is described as either vacuolated or absent [140]. On electron microscopy, the basal layer is largely unaffected, even in severe cases of IEC, but subtle abnormalities in mitochondrial and desmosomal structure are already evident (fig. 27). The ultrastructural pathology becomes progressively more abnormal as keratinocytes move outward towards the granular layer. Mitochondria undergo progressive vacuolar degeneration, leaving perinuclear 'haloes' (fig. 28), and keratin filaments become sparse in the stratum granulosum, leaving a progressively 'empty' cytosol (fig. 29). Desmosomes display a partial loss of internal substructure, with effete, subjacent bundles of attached keratin filaments (fig. 29). Though lamellar bodies form normally, in some cases they appear to aggregate quickly (fig. 30c) and are often secreted prematurely (fig. 30a). Yet, sites with premature secretion can be interspersed with adjacent areas where these organelles fail to be secreted, instead remaining restricted to the peripheral cytosol (fig. 29 and 30b). The latter process correlates again with

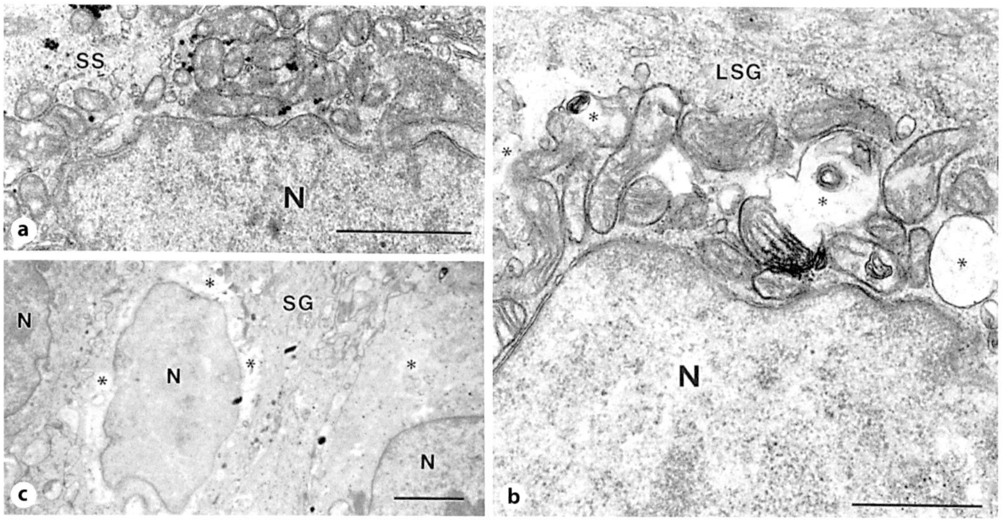

Fig. 28. Progressive mitochondrial degeneration leads to perinuclear vacuolization (from **a** to **c**) in severe IEC (**b**, **c**, asterisks). SS = Stratum spinosum; LSG = lower stratum granulosum; N = nucleus. **a**, **b** Magnification bars = 1 μm. **c** Magnification bar = 2.5 μm.

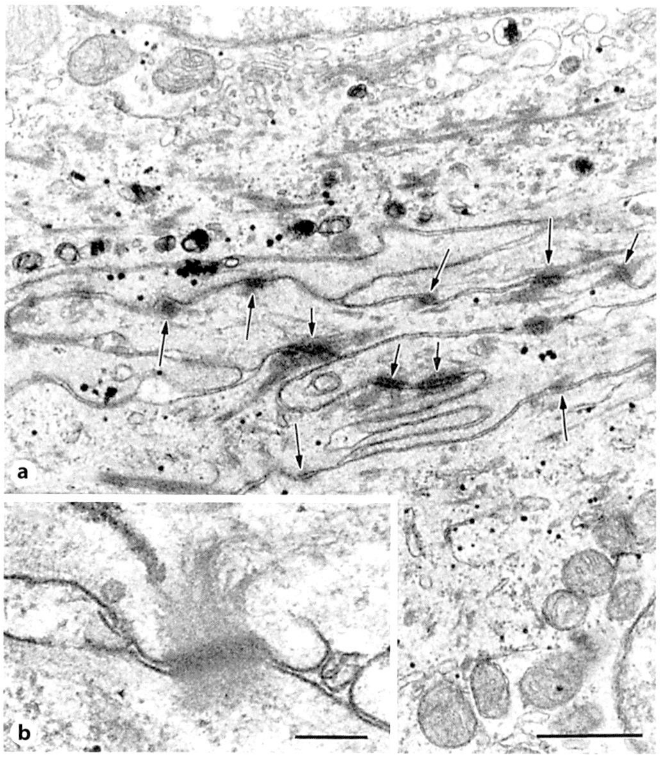

Fig. 29. Lack of keratin filaments and effete desmosomes in IEC. **a** Desmosomes (arrows) appear effete. Short tufts of filaments remain attached to desmosomes, which show no internal structural detail (**b**). **a** Magnification bar = 0.5 μm. **b** Magnification bar = 0.25 μm.

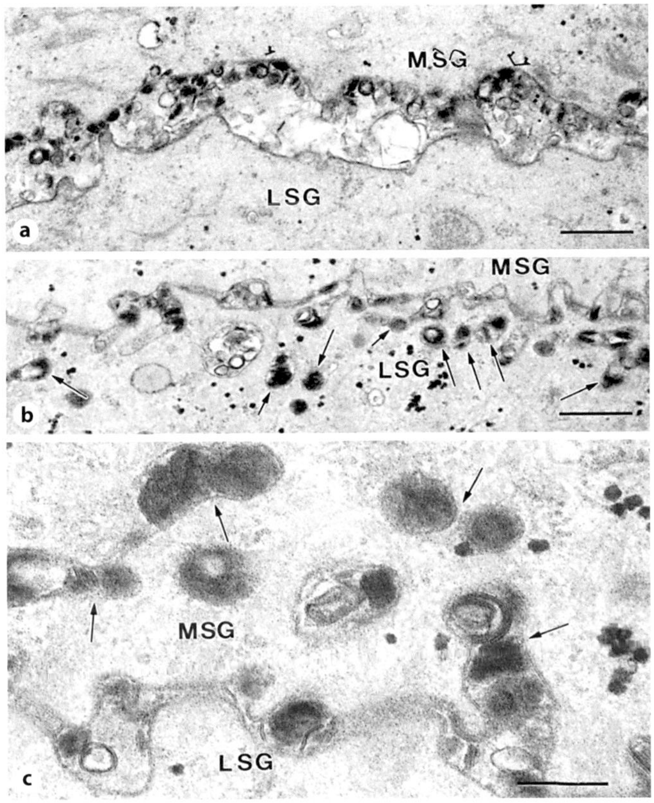

Fig. 30. Abnormal lamellar body secretion in severe IEC. LSG, MSG = Lower, mid stratum granulosum. **a** Lamellar body contents (open arrow) in intercellular spaces in lower-to-mid stratum granulosum. **b** Foci of impaired secretion (arrows) are interspersed with sites of premature secretion (see **a**). **c** Fusion of lamellar bodies (arrows) occurs immediately prior to or concurrent with premature secretion. **a**, **b** Magnification bars = 0.5 µm. **c** Magnification bar = 0.2 µm.

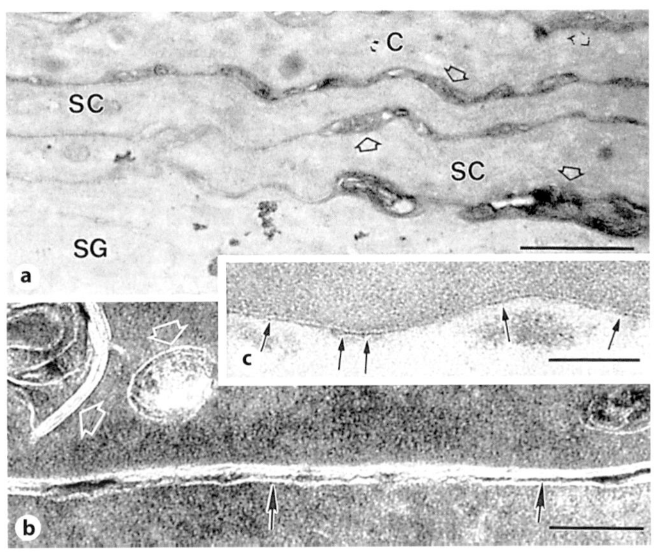

Fig. 31. Paucity of lamellar bilayers, absence of cornified envelopes, absence of corneodesmosomes and entombed lamellar bodies in severe IEC. **a** Delayed processing of secreted lamellar material (open arrows) in lower stratum corneum (SC). SG = Stratum granulosum. **b** Reduced number of lamellar bilayers (arrows) and entombed lamellar body contents (open arrows). **c** Absence of cornified envelopes and corneodesmosomes, but normal corneocyte lipid envelope (arrows). **a** Magnification bar = 1.0 µm. **b**, **c** Magnification bars = 0.1 µm.

the presence of abundant, unsecreted (entombed) lamellar body contents within corneocytes (fig. 31b). Furthermore, there is delayed processing of secreted lipids into mature lamellar bilayers (fig. 31a) and a paucity of lamellar bilayers, even in the outer stratum corneum (fig. 31b). But in some cases, lamellar body secretion is normal, with only processing impaired. Finally, in 3 severely affected patients, there is a striking failure of cornified envelope formation and a lack of corneodesmosomes; in some milder cases, corneodesmosomes and cornified envelopes are normal, and in all cases, the corneocyte lipid envelope appears normal (fig. 31c).

Importantly, all of these features largely normalize in the 'white' ('uninvolved') skin sites of IEC, although keratin filaments remain sparse in suprabasal cells, even in 'uninvolved' skin sites. In summary, the constellation of a near-normal basal layer, surmounted by suprabasal cells with a paucity of keratin filaments, effete desmosomes with or without corneocytes that lack cornified envelopes and corneodesmosomes, is diagnostic of IEC.

4.4. References

1 Hohl D, Williams ML: Ichthyoses and related mendelian disorders of cornification (MEDOC); in Irvine A, Hoger P, Yan A (eds): Textbook of Pediatric Dermatology. In press.
2 Di Giovanna JJ, Bale SJ: Clinical heterogeneity in epidermolytic hyperkeratosis. Arch Dermatol 1994;130:1026–1035.
3 Sahn EE, Weimer CE Jr, Garen PD: Annular epidermolytic ichthyosis: a unique phenotype. J Am Acad Dermatol 1992;27:348–355.
4 Joh GY, Traupe H, Metze D, et al: A novel dinucleotide mutation in keratin 10 in the annular epidermolytic ichthyosis variant of bullous congenital ichthyosiform erythroderma. J Invest Dermatol 1997;108:357–361.
5 Sybert VP, Francis JS, Corden LD, et al: Cyclic ichthyosis with epidermolytic hyperkeratosis: a phenotype conferred by mutations in the 2B domain of keratin K1. Am J Hum Genet 1999;64:732–738.
6 Sprecher E, Ishida-Yamamoto A, Becker OM, et al: Evidence for novel functions of the keratin tail emerging from a mutation causing ichthyosis hystrix. J Invest Dermatol 2001;116:511–519.
7 Fritsch PO: Retinoids in psoriasis and disorders of keratinization. J Am Acad Dermatol 1992;27:S8–S14.
8 Bickenbach JR, Longley MA, Bundman DS, et al: A transgenic mouse model that recapitulates the clinical features of both neonatal and adult forms of the skin disease epidermolytic hyperkeratosis. Differentiation 1996;61:129–139.
9 Rothnagel JA, Dominey AM, Dempsey LD, et al: Mutations in the rod domains of keratins 1 and 10 in epidermolytic hyperkeratosis. Science 1992;257:1128–1130.
10 Cheng J, Syder AJ, Yu QC, Letai A, Paller AS, Fuchs E: The genetic basis of epidermolytic hyperkeratosis: a disorder of differentiation-specific epidermal keratin genes. Cell 1992;70:811–819.
11 Chipev CC, Korge BP, Markova N, et al: A leucine-proline mutation in the H1 subdomain of keratin 1 causes epidermolytic hyperkeratosis. Cell 1992;70:821–828.
12 Chipev CC, Yang JM, Di Giovanna JJ, et al: Preferential sites in keratin 10 that are mutated in epidermolytic hyperkeratosis. Am J Hum Genet 1994;54:179–190.
13 Syder AJ, Yu QC, Paller AS, Giudice G, Pearson R, Fuchs E: Genetic mutations in the *K1* and *K10* genes of patients with epidermolytic hyperkeratosis: correlation between location and disease severity. J Clin Invest 1994;93:1533–1542.
14 McLean WH, Eady RA, Dopping-Hepenstal PJ, et al: Mutations in the rod 1A domain of keratins 1 and 10 in bullous congenital ichthyosiform erythroderma (BCIE). J Invest Dermatol 1994;102:24–30.
15 Yang JM, Nam K, Park KB, et al: A novel H1 mutation in the keratin 1 chain in epidermolytic hyperkeratosis. J Invest Dermatol 1996;107:439–441.
16 Arin MJ, Longley MA, Kuster W, et al: An asparagine to threonine substitution in the 1A domain of keratin 1: a novel mutation that causes epidermolytic hyperkeratosis. Exp Dermatol 1999;8:124–127.

17 Rothnagel JA, Fisher MP, Axtell SM, et al: A mutational hot spot in keratin 10 (KRT 10) in patients with epidermolytic hyperkeratosis. Hum Mol Genet 1993;2:2147–2150.
18 Muller FB, Huber M, Kinaciyan T, et al: A human keratin 10 knockout causes recessive epidermolytic hyperkeratosis. Hum Mol Genet 2006;15:1133–1141.
19 Terheyden P, Grimberg G, Hausser I, et al: Recessive epidermolytic hyperkeratosis caused by a previously unreported termination codon mutation in the keratin 10 gene. J Invest Dermatol 2009;129:2721–2723.
20 Nazzaro V, Ermacora E, Santucci B, Caputo R: Epidermolytic hyperkeratosis: generalized form in children from parents with systematized linear form. Br J Dermatol 1990;122:417–422.
21 Fuchs E, Cleveland DW: A structural scaffolding of intermediate filaments in health and disease. Science 1998;279:514–519.
22 Miller RK, Khuon S, Goldman RD: Dynamics of keratin assembly: exogenous type I keratin rapidly associates with type II keratin in vivo. J Cell Biol 1993;122:123–135.
23 Ming ME, Daryanani HA, Roberts LP, Baden HP, Kvedar JC: Binding of keratin intermediate filaments (K10) to the cornified envelope in mouse epidermis: implications for barrier function. J Invest Dermatol 1994;103:780–784.
24 Steinert PM, Marekov LN: Initiation of assembly of the cell envelope barrier structure of stratified squamous epithelia. Mol Biol Cell 1999;10:4247–4261.
25 Nemes Z, Steinert PM: Bricks and mortar of the epidermal barrier. Exp Mol Med 1999;31:5–19.
26 Steinert PM: The complexity and redundancy of epithelial barrier function. J Cell Biol 2000;151:F5–F8.
27 Anton-Lamprecht I: Genetically induced abnormalities of epidermal differentiation and ultrastructure in ichthyoses and epidermolyses: pathogenesis, heterogeneity, fetal manifestation, and prenatal diagnosis. J Invest Dermatol 1983;81:149s–156s.
28 Wilgram GF, Caulfield JB: An electron microscopic study of epidermolytic hyperkeratosis: with a special note on the keratinosome as the 'fourth' structural factor in the formation of the horny layer. Arch Dermatol 1966;94:127–143.
29 McGowan K, Coulombe PA: The wound repair-associated keratins 6, 16, and 17: insights into the role of intermediate filaments in specifying keratinocyte cytoarchitecture. Subcell Biochem 1998;31: 173–204.
30 Omary MB, Coulombe PA, McLean WH: Intermediate filament proteins and their associated diseases. N Engl J Med 2004;351:2087–2100.
31 Mommers JM, van Rossum MM, van Erp PE, van de Kerkhof PC: Changes in keratin 6 and keratin 10 (co-)expression in lesional and symptomless skin of spreading psoriasis. Dermatology 2000;201:15–20.
32 Reichelt J, Magin TM: Hyperproliferation, induction of c-Myc and 14-3-3sigma, but no cell fragility in keratin-10-null mice. J Cell Sci 2002;115:2639–2650.
33 Ishida-Yamamoto A, McGrath JA, Judge MR, Leigh IM, Lane EB, Eady RA: Selective involvement of keratins K1 and K10 in the cytoskeletal abnormality of epidermolytic hyperkeratosis (bullous congenital ichthyosiform erythroderma). J Invest Dermatol 1992;99:19–26.
34 Virtanen M, Gedde-Dahl T Jr, Mork NJ, Leigh I, Bowden PE, Vahlquist A: Phenotypic/genotypic correlations in patients with epidermolytic hyperkeratosis and the effects of retinoid therapy on keratin expression. Acta Derm Venereol 2001;81: 163–170.
35 Porter RM, Reichelt J, Lunny DP, Magin TM, Lane EB: The relationship between hyperproliferation and epidermal thickening in a mouse model for BCIE. J Invest Dermatol 1998;110:951–957.
36 Reichelt J, Bauer C, Porter R, Lane E, Magin V: Out of balance: consequences of a partial keratin 10 knockout. J Cell Sci 1997;110:2175–2186.
37 Fuchs E, Esteves RA, Coulombe PA: Transgenic mice expressing a mutant keratin 10 gene reveal the likely genetic basis for epidermolytic hyperkeratosis. Proc Natl Acad Sci USA 1992;89:6906–6910.
38 Reichelt J, Bussow H, Grund C, Magin TM: Formation of a normal epidermis supported by increased stability of keratins 5 and 14 in keratin 10 null mice. Mol Biol Cell 2001;12:1557–1568.
39 Schmuth M, Gruber R, Elias PM, Williams M: Ichthyosis update: towards a function-driven model of pathogenesis of the disorders of cornification and the role of corneocyte proteins in these disorders. Adv Dermatol 2007;23:231–256.
40 Schmuth M, Yosipovitch G, Williams ML, et al: Pathogenesis of the permeability barrier abnormality in epidermolytic hyperkeratosis. J Invest Dermatol 2001;117:837–847.
41 Menon GK, Price LF, Bommannan B, Elias PM, Feingold KR: Selective obliteration of the epidermal calcium gradient leads to enhanced lamellar body secretion. J Invest Dermatol 1994;102:789–795.
42 Aunis D, Bader MF: The cytoskeleton as a barrier to exocytosis in secretory cells. J Exp Biol 1988;139: 253–266.
43 Huber M, Rettler I, Bernasconi K, et al: Mutations of keratinocyte transglutaminase in lamellar ichthyosis. Science 1995;267:525–528.

44 Russell LJ, Di Giovanna JJ, Rogers GR, et al: Mutations in the gene for transglutaminase 1 in autosomal recessive lamellar ichthyosis. Nat Genet 1995;9:279–283.

45 Laiho E, Ignatius J, Mikkola H, et al: Transglutaminase 1 mutations in autosomal recessive congenital ichthyosis: private and recurrent mutations in an isolated population. Am J Hum Genet 1997;61:529–538.

46 Akiyama M, Takizawa Y, Kokaji T, Shimizu H: Novel mutations of *TGM1* in a child with congenital ichthyosiform erythroderma. Br J Dermatol 2001;144: 401–407.

47 Fischer J: Autosomal recessive congenital ichthyosis. J Invest Dermatol 2009;129:1319–1321.

48 Williams ML, Elias PM: Heterogeneity in autosomal recessive ichthyosis: clinical and biochemical differentiation of lamellar ichthyosis and nonbullous congenital ichthyosiform erythroderma. Arch Dermatol 1985;121:477–488.

49 Frenk E, de Techtermann F: Self-healing collodion baby: evidence for autosomal recessive inheritance. Pediatr Dermatol 1992;9:95–97.

50 Van Gysel D, Lijnen RL, Moekti SS, de Laat PC, Oranje AP: Collodion baby: a follow-up study of 17 cases. J Eur Acad Dermatol Venereol 2002;16:472–475.

51 Vahlquist A, Bygum A, Ganemo A, et al: Genotypic and clinical spectrum of self-improving collodion ichthyosis: *ALOX12B, ALOXE3,* and *TGM1* mutations in Scandinavian patients. J Invest Dermatol 2010;130:438–443.

52 Raghunath M, Hennies HC, Ahvazi B, et al: Self-healing collodion baby: a dynamic phenotype explained by a particular transglutaminase-1 mutation. J Invest Dermatol 2003;120:224–228.

53 Akiyama M: The pathogenesis of severe congenital ichthyosis of the neonate. J Dermatol Sci 1999;21:96–104.

54 Oji V, Traupe H: Ichthyoses: differential diagnosis and molecular genetics. Eur J Dermatol 2006;16:349–359.

55 Arita K, Jacyk WK, Wessagowit V, et al: The South African 'bathing suit ichthyosis' is a form of lamellar ichthyosis caused by a homozygous missense mutation, p.R315L, in transglutaminase 1. J Invest Dermatol 2007;127:490–493.

56 Aufenvenne K, Oji V, Walker T, et al: Transglutaminase-1 and bathing suit ichthyosis: molecular analysis of gene/environment interactions. J Invest Dermatol 2009;129:2068–2071.

57 Hohl D: Cornified cell envelope. Dermatologica 1990;180:201–211.

58 Greenberg CS, Birckbichler PJ, Rice RH: Transglutaminases: multifunctional cross-linking enzymes that stabilize tissues. Faseb J 1991;5:3071–3077.

59 Steinert PM, Marekov LN: The proteins elafin, filaggrin, keratin intermediate filaments, loricrin, and small proline-rich proteins 1 and 2 are isodipeptide cross-linked components of the human epidermal cornified cell envelope. J Biol Chem 1995;270:17702–17711.

60 Rice RH, Crumrine D, Uchida Y, Gruber R, Elias PM: Structural changes in epidermal scale and appendages as indicators of defective TGM1 activity. Arch Dermatol Res 2005;297:127–133.

61 Hohl D, Huber M, Frenk E: Analysis of the cornified cell envelope in lamellar ichthyosis. Arch Dermatol 1993;129:618–624.

62 Elias PM, Schmuth M, Uchida Y, et al: Basis for the permeability barrier abnormality in lamellar ichthyosis. Exp Dermatol 2002;11:248–256.

63 Choate KA, Medalie DA, Morgan JR, Khavari PA: Corrective gene transfer in the human skin disorder lamellar ichthyosis. Nat Med 1996;2:1263–1267.

64 Kuramoto N, Takizawa T, Takizawa T, et al: Development of ichthyosiform skin compensates for defective permeability barrier function in mice lacking transglutaminase 1. J Clin Invest 2002;109: 243–250.

65 Jeon S, Djian P, Green H: Inability of keratinocytes lacking their specific transglutaminase to form cross-linked envelopes: absence of envelopes as a simple diagnostic test for lamellar ichthyosis. Proc Natl Acad Sci USA 1998;95:687–690.

66 Rice RH, Crumrine D, Hohl D, Munro CS, Elias PM: Cross-linked envelopes in nail plate in lamellar ichthyosis. Br J Dermatol 2003;149:1050–1054.

67 Ghadially R, Williams ML, Hou SY, Elias PM: Membrane structural abnormalities in the stratum corneum of the autosomal recessive ichthyoses. J Invest Dermatol 1992;99:755–763.

68 Lavrijsen AP, Bouwstra JA, Gooris GS, Weerheim A, Bodde HE, Ponec M: Reduced skin barrier function parallels abnormal stratum corneum lipid organization in patients with lamellar ichthyosis. J Invest Dermatol 1995;105:619–624.

69 Lavrijsen AP, Oestmann E, Hermans J, Boddé HE, Vermeer BJ, Ponec M: Barrier function parameters in various keratinization disorders: transepidermal water loss and vascular response to hexyl nicotinate. Br J Dermatol 1993;129:547–553.

70 Paige DG, Morse-Fisher N, Harper JI: Quantification of stratum corneum ceramides and lipid envelope ceramides in the hereditary ichthyoses. Br J Dermatol 1994;131:23–27.

71 Schmuth M, Fluhr JW, Crumrine DC, et al: Structural and functional consequences of loricrin mutations in human loricrin keratoderma (Vohwinkel syndrome with ichthyosis). J Invest Dermatol 2004;122:909–922.

72 Maestrini E, Korge BP, Ocana-Sierra J, et al: A missense mutation in connexin26, D66H, causes mutilating keratoderma with sensorineural deafness (Vohwinkel's syndrome) in three unrelated families. Hum Mol Genet 1999;8:1237–1243.
73 Camisa C, Rossana C: Variant of keratoderma hereditaria mutilans (Vohwinkel's syndrome): treatment with orally administered isotretinoin. Arch Dermatol 1984;120:1323–1328.
74 Camisa C, Hessel A, Rossana C, Parks A: Autosomal dominant keratoderma, ichthyosiform dermatosis and elevated serum beta-glucuronidase. Dermatologica 1988;177:341–347.
75 Korge BP, Ishida-Yamamoto A, Punter C, et al: Loricrin mutation in Vohwinkel's keratoderma is unique to the variant with ichthyosis. J Invest Dermatol 1997;109:604–610.
76 Armstrong DK, McKenna KE, Hughes AE: A novel insertional mutation in loricrin in Vohwinkel's keratoderma. J Invest Dermatol 1998;111:702–704.
77 Takahashi H, Ishida-Yamamoto A, Kishi A, Ohara K, Iizuka H: Loricrin gene mutation in a Japanese patient with Vohwinkel's syndrome. J Dermatol Sci 1999;19:44–47.
78 O'Driscoll J, Muston GC, McGrath JA, Lam HM, Ashworth J, Christiano AM: A recurrent mutation in the loricrin gene underlies the ichthyotic variant of Vohwinkel syndrome. Clin Exp Dermatol 2002; 27:243–246.
79 Matsumoto K, Muto M, Seki S, et al: Loricrin keratoderma: a cause of congenital ichthyosiform erythroderma and collodion baby. Br J Dermatol 2001; 145:657–660.
80 Maestrini E, Monaco AP, McGrath JA, et al: A molecular defect in loricrin, the major component of the cornified cell envelope, underlies Vohwinkel's syndrome. Nat Genet 1996;13:70–77.
81 Mehrel T, Hohl D, Rothnagel JA, et al: Identification of a major keratinocyte cell envelope protein, loricrin. Cell 1990;61:1103–1112.
82 Steven AC, Bisher ME, Roop DR, Steinert PM: Biosynthetic pathways of filaggrin and loricrin – two major proteins expressed by terminally differentiated epidermal keratinocytes. J Struct Biol 1990; 104:150–162.
83 Hohl D, Mehrel T, Lichti U, Turner ML, Roop DR, Steinert PM: Characterization of human loricrin: structure and function of a new class of epidermal cell envelope proteins. J Biol Chem 1991;266:6626–6636.
84 Ishida-Yamamoto A: Loricrin keratoderma: a novel disease entity characterized by nuclear accumulation of mutant loricrin. J Dermatol Sci 2003;31:3–8.
85 Suga Y, Duncan KO, Heald PW, Roop DR: A novel helix termination mutation in keratin 10 in annular epidermolytic ichthyosis, a variant of bullous congenital ichthyosiform erythroderma. J Invest Dermatol 1998;111:1220–1223.
86 Koch PJ, de Viragh PA, Scharer E, et al: Lessons from loricrin-deficient mice: compensatory mechanisms maintaining skin barrier function in the absence of a major cornified envelope protein. J Cell Biol 2000;151:389–400.
87 Wells RS: Ichthyosis. Br Med J 1966;ii:1504–1506.
88 Okano M, Kitano Y, Yoshikawa K, Nakamura T, Matsuzawa Y, Yuasa T: X-linked ichthyosis and ichthyosis vulgaris: comparison of their clinical features based on biochemical analysis. Br J Dermatol 1988;119:777–783.
89 Cuevas-Covarrubias SA, Diaz-Zagoya JC, Rivera-Vega MR, et al: Higher prevalence of X-linked ichthyosis vs ichthyosis vulgaris in Mexico. Int J Dermatol 1999;38:555–556.
90 Fallon PG, Sasaki T, Sandilands A, et al: A homozygous frameshift mutation in the mouse *Flg* gene facilitates enhanced percutaneous allergen priming. Nat Genet 2009;41:602–608.
91 Scharschmidt TC, Man MQ, Hatano Y, et al: Filaggrin deficiency confers a paracellular barrier abnormality that reduces inflammatory thresholds to irritants and haptens. J Allergy Clin Immunol 2009;124:496–506, 506.e1–6.
92 Sandilands A, O'Regan GM, Liao H, et al: Prevalent and rare mutations in the gene encoding filaggrin cause ichthyosis vulgaris and predispose individuals to atopic dermatitis. J Invest Dermatol 2006;126: 1770–1775.
93 Sandilands A, Terron-Kwiatkowski A, Hull PR, et al: Comprehensive analysis of the gene encoding filaggrin uncovers prevalent and rare mutations in ichthyosis vulgaris and atopic eczema. Nat Genet 2007; 39:650–654.
94 Palmer CN, Irvine AD, Terron-Kwiatkowski A, et al: Common loss-of-function variants of the epidermal barrier protein filaggrin are a major predisposing factor for atopic dermatitis. Nat Genet 2006; 38:441–446.
95 Elias PM, Hatano Y, Williams ML: Basis for the barrier abnormality in atopic dermatitis: outside-inside-outside pathogenic mechanisms. J Allergy Clin Immunol 2008;121:1337–1343.
96 Elias PM, Steinhoff M: 'Outside-to-inside' (and now back to 'outside') pathogenic mechanisms in atopic dermatitis. J Invest Dermatol 2008;128:1067–1070.
97 Compton JG, Di Giovanna JJ, Johnston KA, Fleckman P, Bale SJ: Mapping of the associated phenotype of an absent granular layer in ichthyosis vulgaris to the epidermal differentiation complex on chromosome 1. Exp Dermatol 2002;11:518–526.

98 Zhong W, Cui B, Zhang Y, et al: Linkage analysis suggests a locus of ichthyosis vulgaris on 1q22. J Hum Genet 2003;48:390–392.
99 Smith FJ, Irvine AD, Terron-Kwiatkowski A, et al: Loss-of-function mutations in the gene encoding filaggrin cause ichthyosis vulgaris. Nat Genet 2006; 38:337–342.
100 Gruber R, Janecke A, Fauth C, Utermann G, Fritsch PO, Schmuth M: Filaggrin mutations p.R501X and c.2282del4 in ichthyosis vulgaris. Eur J Hum Genet 2007;15:179–184.
101 Nomura T, Sandilands A, Akiyama M, et al: Unique mutations in the filaggrin gene in Japanese patients with ichthyosis vulgaris and atopic dermatitis. J Allergy Clin Immunol 2007;119:434–440.
102 Presland RB: Function of filaggrin and caspase-14 in formation and maintenance of the epithelial barrier function. Dermatol Sin 2009;27:1–14.
103 Sybert VP, Dale BA, Holbrook KA: Ichthyosis vulgaris: identification of a defect in synthesis of filaggrin correlated with an absence of keratohyaline granules. J Invest Dermatol 1985;84:191–194.
104 Seguchi T, Cui CY, Kusuda S, Takahashi M, Aisu K, Tezuka T: Decreased expression of filaggrin in atopic skin. Arch Dermatol Res 1996;288:442–446.
105 Sugiura H, Ebise H, Tazawa T, et al: Large-scale DNA microarray analysis of atopic skin lesions shows overexpression of an epidermal differentiation gene cluster in the alternative pathway and lack of protective gene expression in the cornified envelope. Br J Dermatol 2005;152:146–149.
106 Fleckman P, Brumbaugh S: Absence of the granular layer and keratohyalin define a morphologically distinct subset of individuals with ichthyosis vulgaris. Exp Dermatol 2002;11:327–336.
107 Gan SQ, McBride OW, Idler WW, Markova N, Steinert PM: Organization, structure, and polymorphisms of the human profilaggrin gene. Biochemistry 1990;29:9432–9440.
108 Scharschmidt TC, List K, Grice EA, et al: Matriptase-deficient mice exhibit ichthyotic skin with a selective shift in skin microbiota. J Invest Dermatol 2009; 129:2435–2442.
109 Presland RB, Boggess D, Lewis SP, Hull C, Fleckman P, Sundberg JP: Loss of normal profilaggrin and filaggrin in flaky tail (ft/ft) mice: an animal model for the filaggrin-deficient skin disease ichthyosis vulgaris. J Invest Dermatol 2000;115:1072–1081.
110 Nirunsuksiri W, Zhang SH, Fleckman P: Reduced stability and bi-allelic, coequal expression of profilaggrin mRNA in keratinocytes cultured from subjects with ichthyosis vulgaris. J Invest Dermatol 1998;110:854–861.
111 Baden HP, Roth SI, Goldsmith LA, Baden SB, Lee LD: Keratohyalin protein in disorders of keratinization. J Invest Dermatol 1974;62:411–414.
112 Holbrook KA, Dale BA, Brown KS: Abnormal epidermal keratinization in the repeated epilation mutant mouse. J Cell Biol 1982;92:387–397.
113 Gruber R, Terron-Kwiatkowski A, Sandilands A, et al: Filaggrin mutations in ichthyosis vulgaris. J Invest Dermatol 2006;126:s40.
114 Gruber R, Terron-Kwiatkowski A, Sandilands A, et al: Proximal versus distal filaggrin mutations in ichthyosis vulgaris. J Invest Dermatol 2007;127:S87.
115 Kuechle MK, Thulin CD, Presland RB, Dale BA: Profilaggrin requires both linker and filaggrin peptide sequences to form granules: implications for profilaggrin processing in vivo. J Invest Dermatol 1999;112:843–852.
116 Takahashi M, Tezuka T, Katunuma N: Filaggrin linker segment peptide and cystatin alpha are parts of a complex of the cornified envelope of epidermis. Arch Biochem Biophys 1996;329:123–126.
117 Pearton DJ, Dale BA, Presland RB: Functional analysis of the profilaggrin N-terminal peptide: identification of domains that regulate nuclear and cytoplasmic distribution. J Invest Dermatol 2002; 119:661–669.
118 Fleckman P, Holbrook KA, Dale BA, Sybert VP: Keratinocytes cultured from subjects with ichthyosis vulgaris are phenotypically abnormal. J Invest Dermatol 1987;88:640–645.
119 Rawlings AV, Scott IR, Harding CR Bowser PA: Stratum corneum moisturization at the molecular level. J Invest Dermatol 1994;103:731–741.
120 Scott IR, Harding CR, Barrett JG: Histidine-rich protein of the keratohyalin granules: source of the free amino acids, urocanic acid and pyrrolidone carboxylic acid in the stratum corneum. Biochim Biophys Acta 1982;719:110–117.
121 Nachat R, Mechin MC, Takahara H, et al: Peptidylarginine deiminase isoforms 1–3 are expressed in the epidermis and involved in the deimination of K1 and filaggrin. J Invest Dermatol 2005;124:384–393.
122 Scott IR, Harding CR: Filaggrin breakdown to water binding compounds during development of the rat stratum corneum is controlled by the water activity of the environment. Dev Biol 1986;115:84–92.
123 Williams ML: The ichthyoses – pathogenesis and prenatal diagnosis: a review of recent advances. Pediatr Dermatol 1983;1:1–24.
124 Rawlings AV, Harding CR: Moisturization and skin barrier function. Dermatol Ther 2004;17(suppl 1): 43–48.
125 Katagiri C, Sato J, Nomura J, Denda M: Changes in environmental humidity affect the water-holding property of the stratum corneum and its free amino acid content, and the expression of filaggrin in the epidermis of hairless mice. J Dermatol Sci 2003;31: 29–35.

126 Krien P, Kermici M: Evidence for the existence of a self-regulated enzymatic process within human stratum corneum – an unexpected role for urocanic acid. J Invest Dermatol 2000;115:414–420.
127 Anton-Lamprecht I, Hofbauer M: Ultrastructural distinction of autosomal dominant ichthyosis vulgaris and X-linked recessive ichthyosis. Humangenetik 1972;15:261–264.
128 Schmuth M, Crumrine D, Presland RB, Fleckman P, Fritsch PO, Elias PM: Basis for the epidermal functional abnormalities in granular layer-absent (AGL) vs -present (PGL) ichthyosis vulgaris. J Invest Dermatol 2005;124:A72.
129 Ohman H, Vahlquist A: In vivo studies concerning a pH gradient in human stratum corneum and upper epidermis. Acta Derm Venereol 1994;74:375–379.
130 Hachem JP, Man MQ, Crumrine D, et al: Sustained serine proteases activity by prolonged increase in pH leads to degradation of lipid processing enzymes and profound alterations of barrier function and stratum corneum integrity. J Invest Dermatol 2005;125:510–520.
131 Demerjian M, Hachem JP, Tschachler E, et al: Acute modulations in permeability barrier function regulate epidermal cornification: role of caspase-14 and the protease-activated receptor type 2. Am J Pathol 2008;172:86–97.
132 Briot A, Deraison C, Lacroix M, et al: Kallikrein 5 induces atopic dermatitis-like lesions through PAR2-mediated thymic stromal lymphopoietin expression in Netherton syndrome. J Exp Med 2009;206:1135–1147.
133 Oji V, Seller N, Sandilands A, et al: Ichthyosis vulgaris: novel *FLG* mutations in the German population and high presence of CD1a+ cells in the epidermis of the atopic subgroup. Br J Dermatol 2009;160:771–781.
134 Macheleidt O, Kaiser HW, Sandhoff K: Deficiency of epidermal protein-bound omega-hydroxyceramides in atopic dermatitis. J Invest Dermatol 2002;119:166–173.
135 Brusasco A, Tadini G, Cambiaghi S, Ermacora E, Grimalt R, Caputo R: A case of congenital reticular ichthyosiform erythroderma – ichthyosis 'en confettis'. Dermatology 1994;188:40–45.
136 Choate K, Lu Y, Zhou J, et al: Ichthyosis en confetti is caused by dominant mutations in KRT10 and shows widespread somatic reversion via mitotic recombination. Science, in press.
137 Camenzind M, Harms M, Chavaz P, Saurat JH: Confetti ichthyosis (in French). Ann Dermatol Vénéréol 1984;111:675–676.
138 Krunic AL, Palcesky D, Busbey S, Medenica M: Congenital reticular ichthyosiform erythroderma – ichthyosis variegata: a case report and review of the literature. Acta Derm Venereol 2003;83:36–39.
139 Moskowitz DG, Fowler AJ, Heyman MB, et al: Pathophysiologic basis for growth failure in children with ichthyosis: an evaluation of cutaneous ultrastructure, epidermal permeability barrier function, and energy expenditure. J Pediatr 2004;145:82–92.
140 Hendrix JD Jr, Patterson JW, Greer KE: Skin cancer associated with ichthyosis: the MAUIE syndrome. J Am Acad Dermatol 1997;37:1000–1002.
141 Elbaum DJ, Kurz G, MacDuff M: Increased incidence of cutaneous carcinomas in patients with congenital ichthyosis. J Am Acad Dermatol 1995;33:884–886.

Appendix 1: Ultrastructural and Histochemical Methods

Debra Crumrine

Tissue Preparation

After taking the biopsy, immediately cut off a piece for electron microscopy (EM) and place it into modified Karnovsky's solution (see below). The faster the tissue is transferred to the fixative, the better the subsequent morphology. Further mincing of the tissue into smaller pieces ($\leq 1\ mm^3$) can then be done under a stereomicroscope, while the specimens are immersed in a drop of fixative. For samples destined for ruthenium tetroxide (RuO_4) postfixation, pieces should be minced into oblong strips, with the longest dimension including all layers of skin. This step is critical for subsequent orientation. Since RuO_4 distorts tissue shape, it is important to cut perpendicularly to the stratum corneum (SC)/stratum granulosum (SG) junction. Moreover, RuO_4 does not penetrate deeply into the tissue specimen; hence, it is critical that subsequent thin sectioning does not extend below the level of RuO_4 penetration. Adequacy of RuO_4 postfixation is easily checked in an adjacent, semithin section. If no black is seen at the SC/SG junction at a light microscope level, then there will also be little or no RuO_4 fixation at the EM level. Ideally, the tissue block should be oriented so that the first semithin section incorporates the SC/SG junction (see below). It is not necessary to include full-thickness SC, unless there is a specific interest in the morphology of the outer SC layers (e.g. as in loricrin keratoderma).

Fixation and Tissue Processing Protocols

The preferred *primary fixative* for diagnostic ultrastructure is modified Karnovsky's fixative, prepared as follows: 2% paraformaldehyde and 2% glutaraldehyde in 0.1 M cacodylate buffer, pH 7.3, or 0.1 M phosphate buffer, pH 7.3, containing 0.06% $CaCl_2$. Specimens should be left at room temperature for 1 h and then stored at 4°C for 18–24 h (overnight). Karnovsky's solution is then removed, and samples are rinsed twice with either cacodylate or phosphate buffer. If further processing is not immediately possible, tissue samples can be stored in buffer at 4°C for several weeks.

For *osmium tetroxide (OsO_4) postfixation*, aldehyde-prefixed samples should be split, with some pieces placed in reduced OsO_4, prepared as follows: 1% OsO_4, containing 1.5% K^+ ferrocyanide in 0.1 M cacodylate or 0.1 M phosphate buffer (this mixture is not stable; therefore, mix just before use and, if possible, mix directly on tissue samples). Samples should be OsO_4-postfixed tissues left for 1–2 h at room temperature in the dark in an externally ventilated hood.

Parallel aldehyde-prefixed samples should be *postfixed in RuO_4*, which is invaluable for visualizing the SC extracellular lamellar bilayers. Prepare fixative fresh, because RuO_4 is not stable in air, as follows: 0.25% RuO_4 (from Polysciences Inc.) in 0.1 M cacodylate or 0.1 M phosphate buffer, pH 7.3. Postfix in this solution for 30–45 min at room temperature in the dark in the hood, as for OsO_4 above.

Ideally, the initial aldehyde step should be performed in a *microwave oven* which both shortens processing times and improves subsequent RuO_4 penetration. Fresh biopsies are microwaved in a laboratory microwave oven (Ted Pella Inc.), set at 37°C, as soon as possible after both biopsy and mincing of tissue samples. Microwaving of both the initial and the postfixation steps should be performed for 2.5 min each in an ice bath followed by repeated buffer rinses.

Samples that have been stored in buffer for prolonged periods can also be assessed, but they should first be put into fresh aldehyde fixative and microwaved for 2.5 min, followed by a single buffer rinse. Then, they should be microwaved in the postfixative(s) for another 2.5 min followed by a water rinse. Temperature of the samples can be controlled using an ice bath around the tissue vials. It is critically important at this stage to rinse tissue samples at least 3 times for 5 min each with distilled water after either RuO_4 or OsO_4 postfixation, because otherwise precipitates can form during subsequent ethanol dehydration in preparation for embedding.

Dehydration

During each step of the dehydration process, solutions are removed from the vials containing the specimens with plastic pipettes. It is important that all of the solution is carefully removed before immersion of the specimens in the next ethanol solution. Also note that lower concentrations of ethanol are more critical for successful dehydration than are subsequent, higher ethanol concentrations. The following sequence should be followed: 2 changes of 50% ethanol, 10 min each; 2 changes of 70% ethanol, 10 min each; 2 changes of 95% ethanol, 5 min each; 3 changes of 100% ethanol, 1 min each; 2 changes of propylene oxide, 30 s each; propylene oxide:Epon (1:1), 45 min on rotator with vial caps off; 100% Epon mixture for 20 min in a vacuum, followed by 2 h on rotator, again without caps on vials.

Embedding

Prepare the epoxy embedding resin by mixing the following ingredients (available from Electron Microscopy Sciences, Box 251, Fort Washington, PA 19034, USA, Tel. +1 215 646 1566). DER 736 resin, 48.6 g; nadic methylanhydride, 55.93 g; EM bed 812, 11.53 g; DMP 30, 2 ml. Stir the polymer mixture with a wooden stick until the mixture is homogeneous or use a closed container and shake until mixed well. Embed tissue samples in flat molds, with co-immersed printed labels. When embedding RuO_4-postfixed tissue, the specimens shall be oriented with all layers of the skin, from the SC to the dermis, perpendicularly to the eventual surface that will be ultrathin sectioned. Frequently, the upper (SC) portion of the tissue sample will tend to curve downward below the SG. Therefore, gently tip the tissue face to optimize the likelihood of cutting perpendicularly to the SC/SG junction. Orientation of RuO_4-postfixed samples can be *very difficult*, because of tissue distortion and the very dark color imparted by this compound. Moreover, RuO_4-postfixed tissues can be very brittle. After proper orientation, polymerize samples in the molds at 78°C for 24 h.

Other Ultrastructural Methods

Pyridine Method for Cornified Envelope/Corneocyte Lipid Envelope Visualization

After taking biopsies, immediately mince pieces (to approx. 1 mm^3) and remove as much of the dermis as possible. Then, immerse tissue samples in absolute pyridine at room temperature for 2 h. Pyridine treatment and subsequent processing should always be performed under an evaporative hood, because traces of this toxic solvent remain throughout tissue processing. After pyridine treatment, rinse tissues 3 times for 5 min in either 0.1 M phosphate or 0.1 M cacodylate buffer, pH 7.4, followed by aldehyde fixation and then reduced OsO_4 postfixation as above.

Lanthanum Tracer Perfusion

Prepare an 8% w/v sucrose in 0.05 M Tris buffer (must be used fresh on the same day as the solution is prepared) and slowly adjust the pH to 7.5–7.6 (do not overalkalinize!), because a further pH increase can provoke irreversible precipitation. Mix the 8% lanthanum ($LaNO_3$) solution at a 1:1 volume ratio with the following EM fixative: 2% paraformaldehyde, 2% glutaraldehyde in 0.1 M cacodylate buffer with 0.06% $CaCl_2$.

For penetration studies, immerse tissues in $LaNO_3$ solution for 1 h at room temperature; then remove the $LaNO_3$ solution, and immediately incubate tissues in the aldehyde fixative (as above) for an additional 1 h at room temperature, or overnight at 4°C. Then, rinse twice in 0.1 M cacodylate buffer, prior to postfixation (in reduced OsO_4), followed by a water rinse, ethanol dehydration and embedding, as above.

Lipase Ultrastructural Cytochemistry

Tissue samples are initially fixed in half-strength Karnovsky's solution, using the same EM protocol, except that for optimal results, *fixation must be performed using the microwave technique*. Following fixation, rinse tissue samples 3 times in 0.1 M cacodylate buffer (tissue must be very well rinsed, or enzyme activity will be inhibited by the fixation) and then transfer samples to the incubation medium (see below). Incubations should be performed for either 16–24 h at 37°C or 5 × 30 s in the microwave at 37°C, followed by a further 30 min in a 37°C oven, without microwaving. Incubations should be followed by immersion for 3 min in 2% EDTA in cacodylate buffer at room temperature. Then rinse 3 times in boiled, deionized water and immerse samples in 0.1% lead nitrate in boiled, deionized water for 10 min at room temperature. Rinse 3 times with boiled deionized water and postfix in reduced OsO_4 for 1 h at room temperature in the dark. After postfixation, rinse 3 times in deionized water, dehydrate and embed following the regular EM protocol.

Incubation Medium: 5% Tween 85; 0.2 M Hepes buffer (pH 7.2), and 2.5% sodium taurocholate in 10% aqueous CaCl. *For negative controls*: (1) the same incubation solution without Tween 85; (2) the same incubation solution with added 20 mM quinine chloride (lipase inhibitor), after a 1-hour preincubation in 20 mM quinine chloride in 0.1 M cacodylate buffer; (3) the same solution with the added acid lipase inhibitor tetrahydrolipstatin (20 μM), after a prior 1-hour preincubation in the solution above. To make 20 ml of incubation medium, use 10 ml of 0.4 M Hepes buffer (9.52 g/100 ml water), 1 ml Tween 85, 0.5 g sodium taurocholate and 2 g $CaCl_2$ in 9 ml boiled and precooled deionized water.

Calcium Localization

Fixative

As fixative (store at 4°C up to 4 weeks) use: 0.8 g paraformaldehyde in 10 ml of 2% glutaraldehyde, prepared with deionized H_2O. Warm to 60°C while stirring and then add 2 drops of 1 N KOH. Stir until completely dissolved and clear, and then cool to room temperature. Add 8 ml of 10% glutaraldehyde (1.6 of 50%) and 0.579 g potassium oxalate, and dissolve. Then add 0.56 g sucrose and adjust volume to a total of 40 ml with deionized H_2O.

Postfixation
For postfixation (after storage at room temperature for up to 1 month) use: 2 g potassium pyroantimonate, 75 ml of 0.01 N acetic acid (0.06 ml glacial acetic acid in 100 ml deionized H_2O). Adjust pH to 7.4 with 0.1 N KOH before adding potassium pyroantimonate; heat and stir until dissolved (this step may require some time).

Preparation
Combine 30 ml of this solution with 10 ml of 4% OsO_4. Mix thoroughly and cool on ice. The final solution must be mixed and used fresh. To fix, mince tissues very finely (<0.2 mm) on ice in fixative overnight at 4°C in the dark, or microwave infixative on high power 3 times for 30 s in an ice bath; then continue fixation for 1 h. Transfer tissues to postfixative (OsO_4) and hold on ice in the dark for 2 h. Then, wash tissues with deionized H_2O at pH 10 (use KOH only to adjust pH) on ice for 15 min, place in 50% EtOH, and continue with dehydration and embedding as above.

Oil Red O Staining for Neutral Lipids

Oil red O solution is prepared as follows: 0.7 g Oil red O in 100 ml propylene glycol. Dissolve small amounts at a time and keep stirring. Heat to 100–110°C and stir for 10 min (do not exceed 110°C since a gelatinous suspension will form). Then, filter through Whatman No. 2 filter.

Staining Procedure
(1) Cut frozen sections (6 µm) fresh or after fixation in formalin. Wash sections in deionized water for 2–5 min to remove excess formalin. (2) Dehydrate sections in pure propylene glycol twice for 3–5 min. Agitate solution occasionally. (3) Transfer sections to the staining solution for 5–7 min and agitate sections occasionally (better results at 60°C). (4) Transfer sections to distilled water for 3–5 min, counterstain with hematoxylin for about 20 s and then transfer to a slide. Drain excess water and mount in glycerine-gelatin.

Appendix 2: Glossary of Terminology

Peter M. Elias

Acquired ichthyosis
A noncongenital form of ichthyosis, associated with an underlying malignancy, infection or metabolic/neurological disorder

Collodion membrane
Tight, shiny cast that encases the newborn, which cracks after some time resulting in irregularly branched fissures

Congenital
Disorder is evident at birth or soon thereafter

Congenital ichthyosiform erythroderma (CIE)
Ichthyosis is characterized by generalized erythema

Disorders of cornification (DOC)
Disorders of terminal differentiation affecting all or most of the integument, characterized by scaling and hyperkeratosis

Hyperkeratosis
(1) Histological: increased thickness of the stratum corneum
(2) Clinical: thick and horny skin, but not necessarily accompanied by visible scaling

Hystrix (or hystrix-like)
Spiky (porcupine-quill-like), organized array of spines

Keratoderma
Localized or circumscribed form of hyperkeratosis

Lamellar ichthyosis (LI)
Ichthyosis in which scales tend to be coarse and large (plate-like scales)

Noncongenital
Disorder becomes evident weeks, months or years after birth

Nonsyndromic ichthyosis
(1) Disorder only affects the skin
(2) Primary ichthyosis
(3) Genetic abnormality is expressed phenotypically only in the skin

Scaling
Visible flakes of stratum corneum of variable size, thickness and color

Syndromic ichthyosis
Ichthyosis as part of a multisystem disorder

Appendix 3: Molecular Diagnostic Resources

(Provided by the Ichthyosis Consensus Group)[1]

Country	Name and address of laboratory	Contact	Genes	Comments	Accreditation
Austria	Department of Dermatology Innsbruck Medical University Anichstr. 35 A-6020 Innsbruck Austria	Matthias Schmuth Matthias.schmuth@i-med.ac.at Robert Gruber R.gruber@i-med.ac.at	*FLG, Loricrin, STS*	Research facilities, analysis upon request	No
France	Department of Genetics Necker Hospital for Sick Children, Tour Lavoisier 3rd floor 149 rue de Sèvres 75015 Paris France	Alain Hovnanian alain.hovnanian@inserm.fr Tél: +33 1 40 61 54 44	*SPINK5, FLG, TGM1, ABCA12, ALOXE3, ALOX12B, ICHTHYIN, CYP4F22, K1, K10, K6A, K16, K6B, K17, GJB2, GJB3, GJB4, GJB6, LOR, ATP2A2, ATP2C1*	Routine and research laboratory	Fully affiliated and accreditated for molecular and prenatal diagnosis in patients and families
Germany	Prof. Heiko Traupe Department of Dermatology University Hospital Münster Von-Esmarch-Str. 58 48149 Münster Germany	Heiko Traupe traupeh@mednet.uni-muenster.de Vinzenz Oji ojiv@mednet.uni-muenster.de NIRK referral center: www.netzwerk-ichthyose.de http://www.netzwerk-ichthyose.de/fileadmin/nirk/uploads/technical_information_EN.pdf	*SPINK5,FLG* Through the *Network for ichthyoses and related keratinization disorders* (NIRK) we also offer DNA extraction and analysis in ARCI, KPI, Vörner, EKV, CDPX2, CHILD, and others	Research facilities; analyses upon request	No

[1] This list will be updated from time to time on the following homepage: http://www.netzwerk-ichthyose.de/index.php?id=27&L=1.

Country	Name and address of laboratory	Contact	Genes	Comments	Accreditation
Israel	Laboratory of Molecular Dermatology Department of Dermatology Tel Aviv Sourasky Medical Center 6, Weizmann Street Tel Aviv 64239, Israel	Eli Sprecher Tel: 97236974287 Email: elisp@ tasmc.health.gov.il	*ABCA12, ABHD5, ALOXE3, ALOX12B, CYP4F22, GJB2 GJB6, GJB3, GJB4, ichthyin, K1, K2, K10, K9, K14, K5, LOR, NAP29, SPINK5, ST14, TGM1, PS33B*	Analysis upon request	No
Japan	The First Laboratory, Department of Dermatology Hokkaido University Graduate School of Medicine N15 W7, Kita-ku, Sapporo 060-8638 Japan	Hiroshi Shimizu shimizu@ med.hokudai.ac.jp Masashi Akiyama akiyama@ med.hokudai.ac.jp	*ABCA12, FLG, TGM1, ABHD5, ALDH3A2, K1, K2, K10, GJB2, GJB6, GJB3,GJB4, EBP, LOXE3, ALOX12B, ichthyin, CYP4F22 and LOR*	Research lab	No
Japan	Department of Dermatology and Kurume University Cutaneous Cell Biological Institute, Kurume University School of Medicine, 67 Asahimachi, Kurume, Fukuoka 830-0011 Japan	Takashi Hashimoto hasimot@ med.kurume-u.ac.jp Takahiro Hamada Hamataka@ med.kurume-u.ac.jp Shunpei Fukuda Fukuda_shunpei@ med.kurume-u.ac.jp	*FLG, STS, K1, K2E, K10, TGM1, ABCA12, ALOXE3, ALOX12B, Ichthyin, CYP4F22, XPD, TGM5, SPINK5*	Gene mutation analysis upon request	No
The Netherlands	Experimental Dermatology, Dept. of Dermatology, Maastricht University Medical Center, P Debijelaan 25, 6202 AZ Maastricht The Netherlands	Maurice van Steensel m.van.steensel@ mumc.nl Michel van Geel m.van.gee@ mumc.nl	*FLG, ALOXE3, ALOX12B, ichthyin, TGM1, TGM5, loricrin, GJB2, GJB3, GJB4, GJB6, GJA1, EBP, NSDHL, ABHD5, FATP4*	Research lab	No, but analysis can be repeated in affiliated, accredited lab, if needed

Country	Name and address of laboratory	Contact	Genes	Comments	Accreditation
USA	GeneDx (CLIA-approved molecular diagnostic laboratory) 207 Perry Parkway Gaithersburg, Maryland 20877, USA	genedx@genedx.com Gabriele Richard, MD, FACMG gabi@genedx.com	*ABCA12, ABHD5, ALDH3A2, ALOXE3, ALOX12B, FLG (select mutations) GJB2, GJB6, GJB3, GJB4, ichthyin, K1, K2, K9, K10, SPINK5, STS, TGM1 (deletion testing).* (Key testing is also available for a large number of other disorders of cornification and other genetic skin disorders (see www.genedx.com for a complete test menú).)	Full service diagnostic lab for clinical diagnosis, carrier testing, and prenatal diagnosis. International service.	Fully accredited lab

Subject Index